THERE IS A SOLUTION

THERE IS A SOLUTION

THE TWELVE STEPS
AND TWELVE TRADITIONS
OF PILLS ANONYMOUS

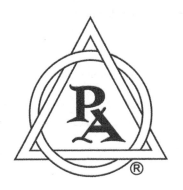

PILLS ANONYMOUS WORLD SERVICES, INC. • CHANDLER, ARIZONA

PILLS ANONYMOUS WORLD SERVICES, INC.
CHANDLER, ARIZONA
Pills Anonymous World Service Office
1900 W. Chandler Blvd., Suite 15-309
Chandler, AZ 85224
info@pillsanonymous.org
www.pillsanonymous.org

ISBN 978-0-9893259-0-5

Pills Anonymous acknowledges and appreciates the text and concepts
of other twelve step organizations shared and/or excerpted herein.

THIS IS P.A. CONFERENCE-APPROVED LITERATURE.

CONTENTS

PREFACE

More Americans now die from drug overdoses than car accidents (Los Angeles Times, September 17, 2011). Painkillers, sedatives, and stimulants now account for more than half of those deaths (Centers for Disease Control, November 4, 2011). Even when the disease of pill addiction does not kill, it destroys the lives of pill addicts, disrupts their families, and wreaks havoc on society as a whole.

There is a solution. Pills Anonymous is based on the premise that pill addicts can recover by helping one another. This idea, of course, did not originate with Pills Anonymous. Other anonymous twelve-step programs such as Alcoholics Anonymous, Narcotics Anonymous, and Cocaine Anonymous have already proved how well this principle works.

Indeed, we are deeply indebted to the twelve-step programs that have come before us and to their members. Pills Anonymous would not have been possible without the extraordinary vision, hard work, and sacrifice of these remarkable people who preceded us. Their efforts to develop and refine the process of recovery have saved countless lives, including our own. Thanks to them, we are no longer harming ourselves, our families, or society. Instead, we lead responsible and productive lives, and try to inspire others to join our ranks. This book is an attempt to express our gratitude for what we have so freely been given.

Pills Anonymous is based on other twelve-step programs but is intended to specifically help pill addicts. When the Pills Anonymous Book Committee was formed, we began by looking at the texts being used by other major twelve-step programs. We then tried to create a combined textbook and study guide specifically designed for pill addicts to use in their recovery.

The result is this book. We hope it will be useful in helping pill addicts to understand the Twelve Steps and Twelve Traditions and apply them in their daily lives. Each chapter explains one of our steps or traditions. Each explanation is followed by one or two short stories written by members of our fellowship. In these stories our members share their personal experience with each step and tradition. Each chapter ends with a list of questions for the reader to answer. This self-examination, which should be done with the help of a fellow pill addict, is central to our process of recovery. We have found a solution for ourselves and have tried to communicate it to others in these pages. We are indebted to the many within the fellowship of Pills Anonymous who contributed to this project. We gratefully dedicate this book to our Higher Power, without whose guidance and inspiration we would have had no chance for success. We pray that our efforts will succeed in delivering a clear message of hope for a new way of life to the pill addict who still suffers. With this book we open our hearts and extend our hands as we welcome you to the fellowship of Pills Anonymous!

— The Book Committee of Pills Anonymous World Services

Twenty Questions

Here are the 20 questions designed to help you determine if you are a pill addict:

1. Has your doctor, spouse or anyone else expressed concern about your use of medications?

2. Have you ever decided to stop taking pills only to find yourself taking them again contrary to your earlier decision?

3. Have you ever felt remorse or concern about taking pills?

4. Has your efficiency or ambition decreased since taking pills?

5. Have you established a supply for purse or pocket or to hide away in case of emergency?

6. Have you ever been treated by a physician or hospital for excessive use of pills (whether or not in combination with other substances)?

7. Have you changed doctors or pharmacies for the purpose of maintaining your supply?

8. Have you received the same medication from two or more physicians or pharmacists at approximately the same time?

9. Have you ever been turned down for a refill?

10. Have you ever taken other peoples pills with or without their permission or obtained them illegally?

11. Have you taken the same pain or sleep medication for a prolonged period of time only to find you still have the same symptoms?

12. Have you ever informed your physician as to which pill works best at which dosage and had them adjust the prescription to your recommendations?

13. Have you increased the dosage, strength or frequency of your pills over the past months or years?

14. Are your pills quite important to you; e.g., do you worry about refills long before running out?

15. Do you become annoyed or uncomfortable when others talk about your use of pills?

16. Have you or anyone else noticed a change of personality when you take your pills, or when you stop taking them?

17. Have you ever taken your medication before you had the associated symptom?

18. Have you ever been embarrassed by your behavior when under the influence of your pills?

19. Do you ever sneak or hide your pills?

20. Do you find it impossible to stop or to go for a prolonged period without your pills?

If you answered yes to three or more of these questions, then our experience would indicate that you may be one of us.

"The Twenty Questions" used in this book have been adapted from the writings of Dr. Paul O. We would like to express our gratitude and appreciation to his family for generously allowing us to use them.

DEFINITION OF PILLS ANONYMOUS

Pills Anonymous is a fellowship of recovering pill addicts throughout the World. The following definition of "Pills Anonymous" will be found in our Fellowship's literature and is often read at meetings of P.A.:

"Pills Anonymous is a fellowship of men and women who share their experience strength and hope with each other that they may solve their common problem and help others to recover from pill addiction. The only requirement for membership is a desire to stop using pills. There are no dues or fees for PA membership; we are self supporting through our own contributions. PA is not affiliated with any religious group, politics, organization or institution. We do not wish to engage in any controversy and neither endorse nor oppose any cause. This is a program which works by regularly attending meetings and working the 12 Steps of Recovery with other pill addicts. Our primary purpose is to carry the message to the addict who still suffers. We work together to stay clean and help others achieve the same freedom."

GENDER DISCLAIMER

Whenever the masculine gender is used in this book in reference to people in general or to a Higher Power, it is to be understood that both men and women are included. This is in keeping with the spiritual principle of anonymity expressed in our Twelfth Tradition, which encourages us to place principles before personalities, and in accordance with our Third and Eleventh Steps, which suggest that we each have a God of our own understanding.

THE TWELVE STEPS OF PILLS ANONYMOUS

1. We admitted we were powerless over our addiction to pills and all other mind-altering substances—that our lives had become unmanageable.

2. Came to believe that a Power greater than ourselves could restore us to sanity.

3. Made a decision to turn our will and our lives over to the care of God, as we understood Him.

4. Made a searching and fearless moral inventory of ourselves.

5. Admitted to God, to ourselves and to another human being the exact nature of our wrongs.

6. Were entirely ready to have God remove all these defects of character.

7. Humbly asked Him to remove our shortcomings.

8. Made a list of all persons we had harmed, and became willing to make amends to them all.

9. Made direct amends to such people wherever possible, except when to do so would injure them or others.

10. Continued to take personal inventory, and when we were wrong promptly admitted it.

11. Sought through prayer and meditation to improve our conscious contact with God, as we understood Him, praying only for knowledge of His will for us and the power to carry that out.

12. Having had a spiritual awakening as the result of these steps, we tried to carry this message to addicts, and to practice these principles in all our affairs.

THE TWELVE STEPS
OF PILLS ANONYMOUS
INTRODUCTION

We come to Pills Anonymous in a state of physical, mental, and spiritual bankruptcy. In the rooms, we find acceptance no matter who we are, what we have done, or where we have come from. By sticking around, attending meetings, and talking with other recovering pill addicts, we find that we share a commonality with people of many diverse backgrounds. Those who might not normally mix or interact have found incredible strength and comfort from the shared experience of active addiction and release from its destructive force. The power of one addict helping another is indisputable, but it is difficult to give to another when our own vessel is drained. Active addiction has taken us to depths of unimaginable despair, corruption, and defeat. Our behaviors and mental obsessions have depleted us of integrity, self-worth, and compassion. We are left with an emptiness that overwhelms us and overshadows all that we do. In order to be of maximum service to others, it would be wise to honor ourselves with much deserved healing. We have found such healing to accelerate and intensify upon acquiring a sponsor and actively working the steps, beginning with Step One and continuing in order through Step Twelve.

When we first embark on honestly working the Twelve Steps, we have surrendered sufficiently to stop using pills and all other mind-altering substances. But we have not yet learned how to deal with life's ups and downs without them. It is a vulnerable place to be, and often a painful place, physically, psychologically, and spiritually. If you are in pain, do not despair; what you are feeling is normal and it does get better. We have found that the sooner we begin working the steps, the sooner we move through the pain of early abstinence into the light of recovery.

Working each step is a two-part endeavor:

1. To gain an understanding of the particular step, what it means, and how it relates to our lives.

2. To make a conscious effort to change our behavior by applying the step in our daily lives.

Contained in the Twelve Steps are principles that we use as defense against the first pill and a return to active addiction. By working the steps we develop our own personal, spiritual toolbox. We learn to rely on, and apply, these tools to life situations and relationships that in the past triggered an uncontrollable compulsion to use. In fact, with continued use, we find the steps and the spiritual principles contained therein to be our survival kit for facing life on life's terms.

The spirit that holds Pills Anonymous together is one of service to the addict who still suffers. We keep what we have by giving it away. We are ill equipped to help another, however, without the tools to perform the job. The wisdom and spiritual principles of the Twelve Steps are powerful tools in assisting us to help one another as suffering and recovering addicts. Any flight attendant will tell us that in the event of an emergency, we are to first put the oxygen mask on our own face and *then* take care of others needing assistance. We have found this to be solid guidance when considering the value of working the Twelve Steps. Although we can share experience, strength, and hope simply by making it into the room of our first Pills Anonymous meeting, the value of our contribution rises in proportion to our commitment and dedication to working the steps. Personal growth from working the Twelve Steps will overflow with abundance to encourage and reassure the fragile newcomer. We find that one of the greatest rewards of helping others work through the steps is that it deepens our own understanding, and we benefit as well.

STEP ONE

"We admitted we were powerless over pills and all other mind-altering substances — that our lives had become unmanageable."

Spiritual Principles: Honesty, Surrender, Acceptance

Step One states our problem. It speaks of our powerlessness, of how our disease has incapacitated us and rendered our lives unmanageable. Taking Step One is an act of surrender that opens the door to the solution available to us in Steps Two through Twelve. The disease of addiction has taken charge of our lives, body and soul. From all appearances, it has destroyed, or at least significantly diminished, our capacity to work, interact, and even love. Our pills possess us. Their importance overshadows all aspects of our lives. Pills have become our constant companion, whether in use or in thought. They supplant relationships, tear up the fabric of our existence, and become the means *and* the end, our lover and faithful friend. The drug, once our "solution," has clearly become our problem.

Power means being able to do or accomplish something. Powerlessness, or having no power, is being unable to achieve or attain a goal. At some point in our use of pills we lost the power of choice and the ability to accomplish the simple act of abstaining from pills or taking them as prescribed. We started prescriptions and told ourselves, "This time I will do it right. I'll make it last," only to find ourselves taking "just two...four...six...ten...more." Some of us started taking pills just to get high and obtained them from friends or from a dealer. The end result was always the same. Shaking an empty pill bottle days later in a panic, we wondered how we would manage until the next refill or score. We lost the ability to act on our own willpower. Many times we told ourselves, "Not today; I am not going to take pills today." Yet, minutes or hours later we found ourselves doing the only thing we could do in order to face the day: we took more pills.

We have lost control. Rationing, limiting our usage to certain times of day, giving our pills to someone else to hold, switching to a different type or strength of pill, switching to a different mind-altering substance, deleting contact phone numbers, switching physicians, and canceling prescriptions are a few of the ways we tried to master control. This list is by no means complete. The fact is, by the time we try to control our pill use we are already out of control. The road of powerlessness takes us to a place where we cannot live with pills, and we cannot live without them. Our pill use controls us.

Addiction affects us in body, mind, and spirit. Our bodies have an allergy that creates an absolute inability to stop using once we begin. One pill can set off an overwhelming craving that must be satisfied. Mentally, we become obsessed with thoughts of using. Everything in our lives takes a back seat when faced with the power of this obsession. The obsession itself appears to have a personality and a will of its own. The isolation and emptiness we experience is the desolation of our spirit. We become detached from everyone and everything—except ourselves and our self-seeking motives and behavior. We have isolated ourselves to the point that pills mean more to us than anything; they have taken over our lives.

Considerable damage has been done to our bodies. Our vital organs have endured unseen abuse. To continue using for some of us will mean organ failure and death. Physically, our nervous systems have become so disrupted and abused that when we stop using, the manifestations of withdrawal are so uncomfortable that it drives us back to using again in order to avoid suffering. Emotionally and mentally, we find ourselves in hell. Inside, we know we are trapped, yet our active disease obscures our vision, telling us our only relief is in a bottle of pills. We find that one is too many and a thousand will never be enough. Ours is a disease of *more*. We will always want more, and once the beast is awakened, it can never be satisfied. There will never be enough. The bottle will always become empty and we will always want more. We are powerless once we take that first pill.

Honesty is essential to recovery. We can no longer live in denial. We tell the truth about our pill use. We tell the truth about our lives. Admitting unmanageability is critical because if we cannot take an honest look at our lives and the wreckage we have created, we will not be willing to change. Change we can and change we must if we are to live a life free of the pain of active addiction. We take a thorough look at our relationships, our home and work commitments, our finances, our health, our spiritual life, our goals and dreams— and we acknowledge how our pill use affected these areas of our lives.

An unmanageable life does not always mean complete failure and a state of utter helplessness. Strained or broken relationships due to complacent, dishonest, manipulative, or emotionally unavailable behavior are an indication of poor management. Isolation from family, friends, and the community in favor of one-on-one time with our pills is a sign that we were not taking care of our innate nature as social beings. Not showing up, coming in late, or using on the job certainly signal an inability to manage our professional lives and careers. Loss of employment from these behaviors qualifies as an extreme example of unmanageability. Depleted bank accounts, unpaid bills, unmet financial obligations, and over-the-top credit card debt from irresponsible spending to support our pill habit and shopping sprees embarked on while under the influence of pills indicate a lack of economic manageability. Legal issues amassed from illegal activities performed in the process of obtaining, selling, and using pills signify an inability to manage life. Hospitalizations for physical ailments related to our pill usage, neglect of those persons in our care, disregard for personal hygiene, lying, broken promises, not taking care of our homes and personal possessions, irresponsible or inconsiderate sexual behavior — these all belong on the list of ways our lives have become unmanageable. Downgrading our abilities, performance, and standards in favor of getting, being, and staying high also qualify for our list. Many of us thought we were managing just fine until we honestly took this step and discovered just how out-of-control our lives had become. In taking this step, we find it helpful to work with a sponsor, another recovering pill addict who has been where we have been and can shine a light on our denial and confusion when we cannot see the truth for ourselves.

Our belief that we can — or might one day be able to — control pills or any mind-altering substance must be destroyed. Denial, rationalization, blaming, minimizing, and justification sprang from our disease and helped to feed it. These strategies also crumbled our ability to see the truth and acknowledge reality. We never forget where we came from. Step One can be revisited any time we start to feel we are back to "normal" and can once again handle a life with pills. Redoing or rereading our First Step is a powerful reminder that we have lost our ability to control, to choose...once we take that first pill.

We cannot build solid recovery on anything less than a firm foundation. Step One is the most important step we take. It is the step of complete surrender. Without complete surrender, we leave room for relapse. We stop fighting. We take this step without reservation, for as long as we think we are in control, we will continue to fight and use. At some point in our using we were blessed with a moment of clarity, a moment of stark realization in which we knew without any doubt that it was too painful to continue on as we had in the past. Pills were no longer working; they were no longer our friend. We were in the grip of a powerful, progressive, incurable disease that if left untreated, would result in our death. For some of us, this window of opportunity — this clarity — came at a low bottom. Others did not have to reach such great depths of destruction and despair. At whatever level we exited the elevator of ruin, with Step One we become willing to do whatever it takes to try a different way of living.

We admit our powerlessness and the unmanageability of our lives. When we admit that we are powerless and cannot successfully manage our own lives, we not only make this admission to ourselves but to others as well. Our admission marks a crucial step toward surrender, but it is acceptance that drives our surrender deeper, inward. When we accept our powerlessness and unmanageability, the information we project out to our world is received back into our hearts and minds as truth and becomes a part of our belief system.

If we have achieved even a small bit of clarity, if the denial which pervades our lives has been chipped away enough so that we can see even the faintest glimmer of light in our desperate existence, then we can see the problem. Our pills are snuffing out the light of our souls.

With the belief that our lives have reached this state of powerlessness and unmanageability, and with the willingness to move forward in recovery, we are ready for Step Two.

OUR MEMBERS' EXPERIENCE WITH STEP ONE

TIRED OF BEING SICK AND TIRED

Admitting I was powerless over my ability to control my use of pills or any other mind-altering substances was painfully simple: I was clearly powerless! My entire life revolved around obtaining, hiding, and using pills. It was a full-time job keeping track of doctors from whom I had obtained prescriptions, DEA prescription-authorization numbers I had stolen, and pharmacists' schedules. Yes, I became a pharmacist stalker! I developed relationships over the phone with a few of them and figured out when the "dumb" ones worked so I could score my pills. I literally had spreadsheets tracking which pharmacies I went to and when.

The amount of work, time, planning, and manipulation that went into my drug addiction consumed every aspect of my life. I think the obsession was even more of a high than actually using the pills themselves. One time when I was starting to withdraw and I was feeling really sick, I called in yet another fraudulent and very illegal prescription. On the way to the pharmacy, I actually began to feel better. Just knowing I would have the pills soon was enough to make me feel high!

My pills always came first. I had three beautiful children under the age of ten and a loving husband of twenty years. I would have stepped over their dead, bleeding bodies to get to my drugs. My disease took a horrific toll on my life. After five years of my lies, cheating, manipulation, and abuse, my husband finally left. I made many promises to stop, always followed by my husband finding my new pill-hiding places or discovering that money was missing from our checking account. I even spent thirty days in an inpatient rehabilitation facility. I went to rehab just to get everybody off my back, and then I relapsed within a month after being released.

My husband left me shortly after that and I still went on for two more horrible years. The pain, fear, and anxiety were overwhelming. My children were in their early teens at this time and wanted nothing to do with me. My husband had found another woman and my parents were disgusted. Finally, one day, after spending 48 hours lying on the bathroom floor, I surrendered. I knew I was completely powerless over my drug addiction and needed help. I called my father and he agreed to call a cab to take me to the airport so I could check myself into a rehab facility that had been suggested by my therapist. I went. I was frightened and beginning to detoxify. Frankly, I was just sick and tired of being sick and tired! I checked myself in and began my journey as a recovering woman.

I completely surrendered and found willingness. I was willing to do whatever it took and I did! Whatever they told me to do I said, "YES." I pushed through the fear. I pushed through the pain. And at the end of sixty amazing days, I found that I had the tools to begin my life of recovery. I have stayed clean for some time since then, and I still attend a meeting every day. I have a sponsor and I sponsor other women. I chair meetings and volunteer to drive women from a halfway house to a meeting once a week. My children are proud of me and have respect for me again. Last week my father told me I was a gift to him and my mother. My husband and I are still apart, but we have found respect for each other and are working on our friendship. Most importantly, I now have respect for myself. I am proud of who I am today and I am eternally grateful that the women in this program have taught me how to live my life as a woman in recovery, with dignity and respect.

"I NEED HELP!"

My addiction reached the point of completely consuming my every thought, emotion, and entire existence. I couldn't live without the pills. In fact, I couldn't do anything without them. They had taken over my entire life. I was failing at every relationship I had. I was definitely in jeopardy of losing my job, and even my freedom. I had done things that were completely against my good judgment and were illegal. I felt lost and stuck, and was sure there was no way out. I never really thought of killing myself, though I took so many pills that there were many times I went to bed thinking I might not wake up the next morning—and that would have been perfectly fine with me.

I was beyond depressed and I spent all my time at home in bed with the blinds drawn. I was high from the moment I woke up until I passed out at night—and the farther gone I could be, the better. I couldn't even get out of bed without rolling over to take my pills first. The addiction was ugly. I was running out of pills more quickly with every passing month, and having to do more and more in order to just keep from being sick from withdrawal. I couldn't live like this any longer, and I didn't have any idea how I was going to stop.

I can remember the day as if it was just yesterday. The images and emotions of that day are still vivid in my mind, which is what I believe keeps me from going back to that way of life. I had been sick in bed, sweating and shaking from head to toe for two days. I had run out of the pain pills I was dependent on, and I couldn't refill my prescription for another twenty-four hours. The pain I felt throughout my body was intense. The withdrawals were unbearable. I suddenly had an overwhelming feeling that there was just no way I could go on one more second without the pills. Immediately following that thought came another: I couldn't imagine putting another one of those pills in my body ever again. I had no idea what to do, but I did know I needed help.

This was the day I surrendered. Step One says, "We admitted we were powerless over our addiction to pills and all other mind-altering substances—that our lives had become unmanageable." This was an understatement for me. My life was completely unmanageable. I ended up calling an addictionologist and told him I needed help. Just like that: I need help. He asked if I could make it to the emergency room, and I told him there was no way I could sit in the ER. I was way too sick. He must have heard in my voice that I was done because this same doctor was not this willing to help me months before. He told me to go to the hospital in an hour and that he would have a room reserved for me to be admitted. So I went! It was hell, but I went. When I got to the hospital, it took them only about an hour from the time I checked in at the desk to the time I was in a bed upstairs in my own room. Thank God, because I honestly don't think I could have put up with more than that.

The next five days I spent in the hospital were filled with a series of shots. I was on such high doses of pills for so long that this was the only way to safely detoxify. And though the shots were definitely no walk in the park, I would do it that way again to manage the horrific withdrawal symptoms. I am grateful that the doctor heard my desperation that day and opted to help me. I honestly think I would have died had I not gotten help when I did. Since that day, I have been willing to do whatever it takes to stay clean. I got a sponsor, made all my follow-up visits with my doctor, and I did service work. I made friends in the fellowship and "stayed in the middle."

Today, after being clean a number of years, my life couldn't be better. I have so much to be grateful for in my life. I notice little miracles every day, and I have wonderful relationships that I thought I had ruined in my active addiction. I have a beautiful relationship with my Higher Power, who I choose to call God, and He enriches my life daily in ways I never knew possible.

I think it is so important that we are thorough when we do Step One. We can't make half-hearted efforts. I've learned that if I work this program, I can find happiness greater than I have ever known. My journey has been a difficult one at times, but I am a better, stronger person because of everything I have endured. Now I have a purpose in life. I love to help other pill addicts. There is no greater gift than to pass on what I have been given.

WORKING STEP ONE

Our healing process must have a beginning, a foundation on which to build our recovery. Answering the questions that follow will, in our experience, help addicts understand the fundamentals and principles of the First Step and give us the solid footing we need as we continue our recovery journey. Our hope is that as we work Step One, the principles will become a part of who we are, and that we will build upon this foundation as we work the steps to come. Reviewing our answers to these questions with our sponsor is an extremely important part of the twelve-step recovery process. A sponsor is a person we ask to help us learn how to work the program of Pills Anonymous. A sponsor should have experience working the steps. Usually of the same gender, a sponsor demonstrates personal characteristics and behaviors we find desirable. A sponsor may be able to give us needed perspective by adding his or her insights based on his or her personal experiences with both addiction and recovery. If you have not asked someone to be your sponsor, now is the time to do so.

1. Was there some specific event or circumstance that created a need for me to start using pills? Explain.

2. How do I feel about the statement, "one is too many, and a thousand is never enough"?

3. Did I ever take pills or other mind-altering substances to change or suppress my feelings? What feelings was I trying to change/suppress? *fear* *fear*

4. What changes in my personality occurred when I was "acting out" in my addiction? (For example: Did I become anxious, self-centered, apathetic, or mean, or passive to the point that I could not protect myself? Controlling and manipulative? Other behaviors?)

5. What changes occurred as my using progressed?

6. When did I come to the realization that my addiction was starting to become a problem? Did I make any effort to change? If so, what did I do to change? If not, why not? *thought I had it under control*

7. In what ways was I manipulative and controlling when it came to getting and using my pills?

8. How have I blamed others for my behavior and my using?

9. To continue my pill use, what things did I do that were completely opposite to my values, principles, and beliefs?

10. How did I feel about myself when I realized I had compromised my values, principles, and beliefs?

11. How did my relationships with myself and others change as a result of my pill use?

12. What legal consequences, if any, have I suffered as the result of my pill use?

13. Have I ever done something that I knew was illegal, something that I could have been arrested for if caught? What were those things? How did I feel about

that at the time? (For example: Did I feel shame? Did I feel smart and proud that I got away with something?)

14. What financial consequences have I suffered as the result of my pill use?

15. What occupational consequences have I suffered as the result of my pill use?

16. What health consequences have I suffered as the result of my pill use?

17. Have I ever had a blackout or passed out as the result of my pill use? Describe the circumstances and results.

18. Have I ever tried to stop using pills and found that I was unable to do so? Did I feel that life was so painful without the pills that I could not stay abstinent very long? Explain.

19. What happened when I ran out of pills? How did I feel and what did I do to get more?

20. What were some of the ways I tried to control or manage my pill use? For example: cutting back on the number taken at one time, spacing the using times farther apart, or switching to other types of pills or another mind-altering substance such as alcohol.

21. Which specific mind-altering substances (including alcohol) have I consumed and abused in the course of my addiction?

22. When my disease was at its worst, what, how much, and how often was I using?

23. When I found myself in a dangerous situation, was I indifferent to the danger or consequences or somehow unable to protect myself as the result of my pill use?

24. How much money have I spent obtaining pills? For example: the cost of the pills themselves obtained from a

pharmacy or other source, doctor or emergency room visits, unnecessary medical procedures, and travel to pharmacies or other countries.

25. Is there some specific event or circumstance in my life that I think I cannot get through clean, one that would prevent me from surrendering to my powerlessness over pills?

26. What will happen to me if I do not address my pill use?

27. Do I think I can still associate with the people, places, and things that were associated with my pill use?

28. What dreams have I discarded, or found myself unable to pursue, as the result of my addiction to pills?

29. What opportunities have I failed to recognize, or have I been aware of, but let pass by as the result of my pill usage?

30. What event or specific events, if any, have brought me to Pills Anonymous?

31. Do I believe that I have a chronic, progressive, and potentially fatal disease? If so, how can I treat it?

This idea was very disappointing to say the least. I knew that I was powerless over my pill use and that my life was chaos in motion, but was spirituality really the answer? Growing up in a spiritually bankrupt home did not give me a head start. I did not have the ability to conceptualize this idea, and it seemed awfully hard to think of going from where I was to believing in God or a power greater than myself. After all, if there was this power, why was I an addict in the first place? It seemed that everyone around me had his or her God or Higher Power, except me. I never believed I could find what those people had. I saw laughter and happiness all around and I wanted that back in my life. I was still very skeptical about the program if spirituality was a necessary component, but I had no place else to go.

It was at that moment that I decided to do the opposite of what my addict brain told me to do. I had listened too long to those thoughts and they led me to nothing but unmanageability and insanity. My relationship with my husband and three children was falling apart, and I had isolated myself from the world and everything in it. I no longer found joy in anything. I had been to treatment and detox centers. Nothing was working. I felt total despair. It was hard to think back to the last time I cared about anything but getting and using pills. I knew that my way of dealing with life was not working. It was then that I became *willing* to believe that the people in the meeting had some answers for me. I had nothing else to believe in. It became clear to me that left to my own devices, I would use pills.

When I was using, I had promised myself after every pill bottle that I was finished. I really meant it, but I ended up breaking that promise to myself time after time. During my first week of recovery, when I felt the compulsion to use pills, I would turn it over to this Higher Power I didn't believe in. My first inkling that there might be something out there helping me was when this turning-over process helped me stop using pills for a week. It certainly was not by my efforts alone that I was staying clean. Forces greater than me were allowing me to not use pills, one day at a time. I then began using this Higher Power in other aspects of my life. If my husband or children made comments about past usage, I would turn that over as well, but I was still skeptical.

I decided to listen to the suggestions of the people who had a lot of clean time, the very ones who had what I wanted. I chose a sponsor I trusted, and started working the steps. The First Step was easy. I knew that pills ruled my life and that my life was unraveling. But I had a problem with the idea of accepting a Higher Power. When I presented my spirituality dilemma to my sponsor, she told me that by doing the steps, going to meetings, and working with others, I would come to understand what everyone was talking about. She claimed that I, too, would believe that a power greater than me could restore me to sanity. I still had concerns about the program, but I knew that I could not go back to the roller coaster my life had become, and that someone or something other than me was keeping me clean.

So began my spiritual journey. Willingness and open-mindedness were necessary companions. My way wasn't working. Maybe, just maybe, hers would. My sponsor explained that Pills Anonymous was made up of many different belief systems. Some were agnostic, atheist, or had lost the faith they once had. I wanted the serenity that came along with spirituality and if a power greater than myself could restore me to sanity, I was more than willing to try to believe what I had not before.

I began to pray, even though it felt unnatural. I asked my Higher Power to show me how to get to where I needed to be in order to remain clean and have serenity in my life. Slowly I developed hope and gained some peace. I hadn't felt those emotions in such a long time, and it felt wonderful!

Guilt and fear were replaced by serenity and sanity. It was working.

Today I realize that I used my sponsor as my Higher Power until I could conceptualize my own. I now talk to my Higher Power on a daily basis. When I am in a confusing or emotional situation, I stop and ask for help, and then I wait for the answers. They always come if I stay connected to the program of Pills Anonymous. I don't know how or why it works so well, but today I don't have to know why. It just works.

Now I Have a Solution

In the moment that I understood the concept of Step Two, I found the open-mindedness I needed to move forward in my recovery. I had been wallowing in self-pity and shame, centered on my admission of powerlessness and unmanageability for months and months, with seemingly no solution until that moment. When I finally heard a definition of sanity that made sense to me, I felt like I could actually admit that I had been insane for years.

I was living in a twenty-eight-day rehabilitation facility after a series of hospital visits, car accidents, and several pain-pill overdoses. I was sitting in a group therapy session when the counselor said a few simple, yet poignant words. He said that insanity is doing the same thing over and over again, expecting different results. That's when Step Two struck me right between the eyes. It was the first time in a long time that I saw things as they really were! I then realized and admitted that I had been completely and utterly insane. My mind flashed on countless memories: Going to the ATM with hopes that all the money wouldn't go to pills, trips to pharmacies with plans not to take all the pills within the first night, numerous doctor visits in which I lied through my teeth to get another prescription. All of those situations ended the same way—disappointment, guilt, and shame. I looked around the room of fellow addicts and felt a moment of complete defeat, finally realizing how insane I had, in fact, been for these years.

The good news quickly followed. The counselor reminded us that Step Two allows us to find or connect with a higher power of our own individual understanding that will help restore us to sanity. Now, I wasn't quite sure that I had ever been sane, but I felt a glimmer of hope from that promise. Knowing what *insanity* looked like, I was interested in what *sanity* was. The counselor informed me that sanity meant having soundness of mind. Oh what a bright vista! I had been trying to chemically induce a state of mental blankness for years! The mere idea of having soundness of mind was incomprehensible, as in the past I had only known terror, bewilderment, and fear.

I've heard in meetings that the concept behind Step Two is hope, and this has resonated with me on several occasions over the years. In early recovery I was given hope that a God of my understanding would restore me to sanity, and I'd be able to live without daily use of copious amounts of pain pills. That promise came through as a result of getting a sponsor and working the remaining steps of the program. In the last several years, I've seen the God of my understanding restore me to sanity in dealing with many aspects of my life. As an addict, sanity doesn't always come naturally and instinctively, but now I have a solution that has worked in the past and that works when I use the simple set of tools available through the Twelve Steps. To get back to sanity, I know what works: keeping close to the program, staying honest with a sponsor, and being open-minded about letting God restore me to sanity. To me, understanding Step Two paves the way for the next ten steps, which require fearless action. I truly believe that having faith in a God of my understanding made it possible for me to approach those remaining steps.

Working Step Two

After finishing Step One and discovering the insanity of our disease, we will need the hope that Step Two brings to our recovery. Answering the following questions with the help of a sponsor will assist us in understanding and embracing the fundamental principles given to us in Step Two.

1. Based on the definition of sanity discussed in this chapter, what are some examples of my behavior that are contrary to this definition? For example: Did I often not act in the best interests of myself or others? Did I try to control my pill use? Did I put myself or others in dangerous situations? Did I quit jobs, friendships, or other relationships because they interfered with my pill use? Did I physically injure myself or others? Did I ignore real medical issues because I was afraid my pill usage would be discovered?

2. For each of these examples, what would have been the sane thing to do?

3. Finding myself able to do something sane even one time in a circumstance or situation where I was not able to in the past can be considered evidence of sanity. Have I had any experiences like that in my recovery? What were they and what do I think led me to act sanely?

4. In what areas of my life do I need sanity now?

5. What concepts of a Higher Power was I taught as a child?

6. What is my current concept of a Higher Power?

7. What do I want to believe about a Higher Power?

8. What fears do I have about "coming to believe"?

9. Do I have problems accepting that there is a power greater than myself?

10. What is holding me back from acceptance of such a power? (For example: fears, inability to trust, and ego).

11. Have I ever believed something for which no real physical evidence existed? What was the experience like?

12. Have I asked for help from my sponsor, gone to meetings, and reached out to other recovering pill addicts? What were the results?

13. What experiences shared by other recovering pill addicts about "coming to believe" have I connected with? Have I tried to incorporate any of them into my thinking and my life?

14. Why is having a closed mind dangerous to my recovery? How can I demonstrate open-mindedness in my recovery and my life today?

15. Am I willing to acknowledge the possibility that a Higher Power of my own understanding could restore me to sane behavior?

STEP THREE

"Made a decision to turn our will and our lives over to the care of God as we understood Him."

Spiritual Principles: Willingness, Faith, Surrender

Step Three challenges our level of commitment to recovery. Are we willing to go to any lengths to remain clean and to learn a different way to live? For years we have run our lives with iron-fisted control. The very idea of relinquishing command can be at once absurd and frightening. Step Two opened a window in our resistant psyches to the possibility of accepting help from a power greater than our own. Step Three is where we turn our new, perhaps delicate, belief into action by making a decision.

When breaking down Step Three, we see it has several parts. First, we make a decision. Next, we determine what constitutes our will and our lives. Finally, we seek an understanding of God by placing our will and our lives in God's care. Looking at the meaning of three important words may be helpful to understanding this step. The act of making up one's mind is a *decision*. *Will* is the mental faculty we use to deliberately choose or decide upon a course of action. *Care*, in

31

this context, means supervision, or protection. When we re-read Step Three in the context of these definitions, it takes on new meaning for many of us. Unless we make up our mind and conclude that we need help, we do not have a chance at recovery. Our will, unaided, has led us down some very unhealthy paths. We have made many damaging decisions on our own, over and over again. In light of our track record, it makes more than a little sense that we would benefit from some "supervision and protection"!

A couple of myths about Step Three often block pill addicts from making this critical commitment.

MYTH #1: We have to feel as if we are completely and totally in contact with our Higher Power, almost as if we are expected to have a profound spiritual experience, in order to complete this step.

FACT: We are not seeking perfection with this step. We are making a decision—just a decision—to begin the process of relinquishing control. And as we continue thoroughly working through the steps, we begin to experience a spiritual awakening.

MYTH #2: The use of the word "God," and even the gender "Him," have some religious connotation or sexual bias.

FACT: We are simply maintaining a tradition established by the inspired men and women who launched Alcoholics Anonymous. You can call *your* Higher Power anything you want, and refer to that power as him, her, it, or any other term you wish. You will find, in most twelve-step fellowships that "God" is merely a "common denominator" we use to refer to our respective Higher Powers.

Step Three is but a beginning in a journey of spiritual growth. We do not need a definition of God to proceed. In fact, we may never have a clear definition of our Higher Power. What we will have, and what we will continue to develop, is an awareness and understanding of a power greater than ourselves. We begin to realize and experience that we are not alone. Steps Four through Twelve will continue to teach us and help us develop our understanding of God. As we level our pride, become accountable, and perform acts of service, we begin to acquire a sense of what our Higher Power means to us. For now, we need the willingness and open-mindedness to investigate without prejudice or preconceived judgment.

We find that intolerance to spiritual principles is an obstacle to recovery. Patience and willingness will melt the most solid block of indifference. As we sit in a meeting of Pills Anonymous, we can look around the room and see others who have taken Step Three. By listening to them share their experience, strength, and hope we learn that they have come to rely on the God of their understanding to guide their decisions and their lives. When listening to the gut-level honesty of another recovering pill addict, it is difficult to continue to deny or doubt the power of God, in whatever way we may understand that power. Sometimes slowly, but always surely, we begin to see that God works. We may first see the manifestation in others as they describe positive events and shifts in perception that prior to working the steps had seemed unimaginable or unattainable. What becomes more clear to us as we stay the course in recovery is that there is a power that does for us what we cannot do for ourselves *if* we remain open to it.

At this point in our recovery, we can look back at Step One with honest reflection. If we are truthful, we recognize that when we ran the show, our results were less than desirable. Step Three is our opportunity to try something different. We can stop running the show and surrender the burden of control. We no longer have to keep running up against life, in constant collision with people, places, and conditions. We can stop struggling and stop fighting.

Step Three does not mean that we now just sit back and let life happen without active participation. We are still responsible for action. The difference is that we are no longer acting as sole director of the universe. We give up the driver's seat. We actively work on developing a relationship and open communication with the Higher Power of our understanding. We ask for guidance to do the next right thing, rather than acting on our own impulse. When we find ourselves wandering off on our own authority, we simply come back to this step and renew our commitment.

Step Three also does not mean we will now live a life of complete ease and comfort. Life happens on life's terms. We remain an integral part of humanity. The road will continue to have steep inclines, muddy passages, blind corners, and dead ends. Many of us have experienced some of our most painful life circumstances in recovery, and we have found that we can stay clean even through the most challenging times. No longer operating on our own power has allowed us new insight and perspective that provides courage and healing. The ability to face and walk through fear and loss without picking up pills to help us cope has strengthened our respect for, and commitment to, Step Three.

The following is a simple Third Step prayer that captures the essence of the Third Step's meaning, helping us to remain open and willing:

> God, I place my will and my life in Your care.
> Open my mind and my heart to the light of Your guidance.

With every positive stride we make in our recovery, we are building spiritual muscle. Every time we surrender our pride and make a willing, open invitation to our Higher Power to enter our mind and heart, we are forging a pathway and strengthening the connection. What may once have seemed impossible to achieve, will one day be accomplished as effortlessly as breathing. With firm ground beneath us and a loving Power surrounding us, we move on to Step Four.

OUR MEMBERS' EXPERIENCE WITH STEP THREE

THE CRITICAL LINK

It wasn't until after I had suffered my third relapse with pills that I finally came to understand my biggest problem in staying clean: I was not fully grasping and accepting the Third Step. Every time I stopped using and got a little bit of recovery under my belt, it was only a matter of time until I experienced the powerful compulsion to step out and run my own life again. Even though I had no problem (initially) turning my will and my life over, the fragile spiritual connection I had carefully managed to reestablish with my Higher Power after years of self-abuse quickly faded away as I gave in to the overwhelming temptations of ego and stubborn self-will.

The pressure and demands of daily living, work, family, and routine began to slowly chip away at my serenity, and at my program of recovery. As I began to lose myself (once again) to these trivial challenges, I also lost my perspective. Instead of embracing the safety and fellowship available to me in the rooms, I started to flee in the opposite direction, abandoning all of the tactics that had saved me in the first place!

The first things to go, it seems, were always prayer and meditation. I suddenly couldn't seem to find or make time to communicate with my Higher Power anymore. When this critical link collapsed, it was all downhill from that point. I stopped calling my sponsor. My attendance at meetings tapered off, and then finally stopped altogether. I was no longer connected with the vital, spiritual force of the fellowship and the guiding principles that made my continuing recovery possible.

I noticed subtle changes in myself. Anger, jealousy, and resentments began to creep back in, poisoning my relationships with others. I became increasingly closed-minded, and extremely negative in my thinking. I seemed to be, once again, returning to that previous state of living "almost at the animal level." From this point, it was only a matter of time until I would make that first call, and start using pills again.

Returning to the rooms of recovery again after a third relapse was one of the hardest things I've ever had to do. I was consumed with fear, self-pity, and self-loathing. I honestly didn't know if I was going to be able to successfully stay clean this time, but I also knew that I had to give it my absolute best effort. The last run had ruined my health, unhinged my sanity, and very nearly killed me, and I had no illusions about where I would end up if I relapsed one more time. If I used again, they might as well start preparing the headstone, because I'd be needing it very soon!

Also, my poor, long-suffering wife of many years had finally come to the point where she could no longer take any more, either. She let me know, in no uncertain terms, that if I started using again, she would have to let me go, because she couldn't bear to watch me destroy myself anymore. I knew she meant it, and I couldn't blame her. Additionally, I had become so debilitated from my drug use that I was unemployed and unemployable. The wreckage was monumental, it seemed.

But I was fortunate in one way because I knew there was still a solution. I could, even now, pick up the pieces of my shattered life if I could manage to somehow restore my connection with my Higher Power, return to the rooms, and try to keep doing "the next right thing" one day at a time. The key to my salvation has turned out to be quite simple, actually. I've discovered that the best way for me to achieve happiness and peace of mind is by helping others, and trying to be of service.

I do my best now to maintain a daily routine that includes time for prayer and meditation because I've found that this provides the peace of mind and serenity that I cannot live without. Today, I have to remember to practice the Third Step every single day. It's the only way I can maintain my sanity and my focus on what matters most in life. It's when I find myself under the greatest stress and strain that I must remember to turn my will and my life over. This can prove to be a tremendous relief at times, because while *I* may not always have the answers, *my Higher Power* certainly does. And I find that the direction is always there if I'm listening carefully. As long as I can remember to keep following this plan, I feel I'll continue to stay clean and lead a good life, filled with purpose and reward.

MY WAY MADE ME MISERABLE

When I came into P.A., I was desperate to stop using pills. I had tried time and time again to quit, but I just couldn't. I felt like a total failure. What was wrong with me? Why couldn't I just stop? I felt completely hopeless. Who could possibly help someone like me?

But a day did come, as I stood sobbing at my kitchen sink, when I cried out to God for help. I begged Him to stop me from using pills because I couldn't do it on my own. And He made it so. I found myself in a treatment program, with the willingness to do what was suggested to me. In the beginning I was told I should get a sponsor. I was told to call people in the program. I was told to go to meetings. And I was told to start doing the steps. I didn't know why I was doing these things, but it didn't matter. All I knew was that something had to change because when I did things my way I was miserable. So I gave it a try. I began turning my will and my life over to the care of God and the program, and basically just did what was suggested. And what everyone had said was right: Life started getting better, things became easier, and the promises began coming true.

But it wasn't long before the addict in my head began talking to me again, and soon I found myself battling old behaviors. When I had a bad day, my head would tell me not to call my sponsor or anyone else because I didn't want to "bother them" or that "I was just being stupid, and it would pass." And when women at my job started talking to me about how they were taking pills to survive at work, and it really made me uncomfortable, I kept it inside and told myself that it wasn't a big deal. When something bothered me, I held it inside and let it fester instead of asking God and my sponsor for help. And slowly, I began to replace the positive things my program had taught me with the negative things my addiction was telling me. Before I knew it, I had convinced myself that I was "fine" and that I could run the show again.

So, I began skimping on meetings. I rarely called my sponsor, and when I did call, it would be to convince her that everything was "fine." I even did some step work just so I could say I was doing the steps, but in reality I had mentally begun to check out of my program. I stopped putting God and my program first and tried doing things my way, but once again I was reminded that my way made me miserable.

One day at work a coworker took out a pretty, shiny box from her purse and flashed me her "happy pills" as she called them. Without even thinking I took one, popped it in my mouth, and swallowed fast. Being in shock at what I had just done I thought about throwing it back up, but I couldn't. So, I went along for the ride, and by that night I had started drinking again because I didn't like the feeling of the pill wearing off. The next day I was back at work, digging through my coworker's purse and popping another pill, then spending the entire day miserable; paranoid that someone was going to know and I was going to lose my job. So, after only a couple days of experiencing that once dreaded misery, I knew I didn't want to go back to that life. I cried out to God for help again. He gave me the courage to tell my husband what I did, and then He gave me the strength to go to a P.A. meeting that night and admit that I had relapsed. I got myself back into the program and gave it my all.

What I have learned is that when I turn my will and my life over to God and my program, and do what is suggested of me, life gets better. And when I listen to God, and not the addict in my head that wants to take me down, I feel better. Today I wake up each morning with a thank you to God for how far I've come in my recovery, and then I pray for His will to be done and not my own, for I know that when I am in control I am miserable , and when God is in control I am happy.

WORKING STEP THREE

Deciding to turn our will and our lives over to the care of God—or anyone else—is a huge leap of faith and not an easy task. With our surrender from Step One and the hope we received from Step Two well in hand, we are able to demonstrate our willingness to try another approach in our lives. Many of us have consulted with our sponsors in answering the following questions in order to help us make, quite possibly, the most important decision of our lives.

1. Why is making a decision essential to working this step? Can I make this decision just for today, one day at a time, or for one hour at a time?

2. Do I have fears about making this decision? What are they?

3. What areas of my life do I believe are difficult to turn over to my Higher Power?

4. In what ways has my self-will been ineffective in managing my life, and how has self-will hurt me, as well as others?

5. Were there times, such as when I wanted to stop using pills, that my own will or willpower was insufficient?

6. What is my current understanding of "God," or a "power greater than myself," and how is that power working in my recovery and my life today?

7. Am I beginning to recognize the difference between the things I can change and the things I cannot? What are some examples of the things I can change? What are some examples of the things I cannot change?

8. Am I willing to turn the things I cannot change over to the care of my Higher Power?

9. Am I willing to ask for help in order to take care of myself and others?

10. How have hope, faith, and trust become positive forces in my life today? What further actions can I take to further develop and apply these principles in my life as my recovery progresses?

11. What actions do I plan to take to follow through on the decision I made in working this step?

STEP FOUR

"Made a searching and fearless moral inventory of ourselves."

Spiritual Principles: Honesty, Courage

Many of us have a tendency to be great starters. We pick up projects, relationships, jobs, and new ideas with much enthusiasm. But when the going gets rough, dull, or simply inconvenient, we quickly lose our motivation to follow through, and often drop the ball. Promises made in the heat of the moment, when emotions run high, are ditched at the first sign of reality or struggle. We do not want to repeat this habit with our recovery.

Anytime complacency, fear, or doubt set in, we can look back at Step One and remember what brought us to our bottom in desperation. Broken and shaking, we walked through the doors of a Pills Anonymous meeting. We met people just like us and listened as they shared their stories. We found similarities in their experiences and received a spark of hope. We developed a desire to build on this newfound promise of a better life. If we have been sincere and thorough, we have hung on to our recovery—our oasis in the desert—for dear life. As we travel farther into our recovery, it is important to express to our sponsor any doubts or fears we may have. We do not hang on to these thoughts and emotions alone, for they are the fuel we may use to "cut and run" before we experience all the miracles of recovery. Fellow pill addicts who have taken Step Four before us are familiar with the angst and uncertainty we feel when facing this step.

Step Four is the part of our program where we start to clean house—our house. This may be the first time for many of us to take an honest look at our lives. What is this big unknown called a "moral inventory"? We start by simply listing our personal assets and liabilities, what helped us and what held us back, what empowered us and what kept us stuck. We look at the beliefs, motivations, compulsive tendencies, and behavior patterns that ruled and directed our lives. We shine the light on who we are and who we have been. Our recovery depends on more than abstinence from pills and other mind-altering substances. We have found that we need a profound change in our thinking and actions. We cannot seek help to change what we do not know or cannot see. Step Four is our opportunity to learn about ourselves and our lives. We can keep whatever will serve our recovery, and seek God's help in changing, or letting go of, anything that does not.

Many of us have been reluctant to start this step because we were afraid of what would be revealed. Some of us were eager to get it over with, hoping to find relief from the mental burdens and emotional pain of the past. Whatever the case, it should help to know that this step, like all the steps, is not taken alone. Our sponsor is an invaluable asset when working this step; communication with him or her will ease our anxiety and confusion. Having walked this road before us, our sponsor has an uncanny knack of knowing what to say to encourage us to persist when we feel frustrated. We also remember we have opened up to a power greater than ourselves in Steps Two and Three. Our Higher Power is available to help us when doing our inventory. All we have to do is ask for guidance. As we sit down to think about or write out our Fourth Step, we ask the God of our understanding to remove any fears or defenses we have that may keep us from looking at the truth about our lives. We ask for the courage to remember and see clearly what we need to include in our inventory.

Step Four is vital to our recovery, so we take our time, but once we have started, we avoid procrastination. We put pen to paper or fingers to keyboard and continue as best we can until completion. We do not worry about doing this step perfectly. We want to be as honest and thorough as we can at this time in our recovery. We have spent our whole lives developing and fine-tuning our character defects. It may be hard to detect what we need to change at first glance. Self-righteousness and self-justification can be sly and subtle foes when working this step. We remember to keep the focus on ourselves and on our behavior. Blaming others keeps us in the shadows. We are ready to walk out of the darkness, free from the bondage of our past. We take care to focus on our side of the street. To do this, we must be vigilant and take responsibility only for ourselves.

Our inventory will not be complete without including our assets—those parts of us that we consider strengths. Acknowledging our positive qualities, characteristics, and abilities is equally important to our recovery. Our inherent nature is a pure and loving spirit. Recovery and the steps guide us back to the truth about our inner self. We may have deserted many of our dreams and ambitions in the midst of our active addiction. Recalling our unrealized hopes and aspirations as we work this step may help us realize that, with recovery, our lives can once again hold wonderful possibilities.

As we continue in recovery, we gain a clarity and perspective that eluded us in the early days of our recovery. More *will* be revealed. When that happens, we revisit Step Four and dig deeper. We stay clean one day at a time, yet our recovery is a journey, and the Fourth Step is one of discovery and freedom. We grow into deeper and deeper levels of understanding about ourselves. Step Four is the beginning of a relationship, one we have neglected for a long time: the relationship we have with ourselves.

OUR MEMBERS' EXPERIENCE WITH STEP FOUR

SEARCHING, FEARLESS, AND THOROUGH

As I came to Step Four, it seemed like it shouldn't be that big of a deal; yet I often heard that many people relapsed while on this step. Relapse may be a part of most people's stories, but I didn't want it to be a part of mine. So right after my work was done on the Third Step and I had developed a relationship with a definitive Higher Power, I started right away on my Fourth Step. However, as it turned out, my version of "right away" was not as fast as I had hoped. I began to see why some addicts never completed this step. I would sit down in a quiet place and thoughts of all the terrible things I had done overwhelmed me. It felt like too much to bear, so I put it off, always saying I would return to it the next day. Before I knew it, a month had passed.

My sponsor had warned me that this might happen. It is difficult to face the bottled emotions we know are going to flow out. My sponsor, who has been clean for many years, knows what he is talking about, and I needed to accept his guidance. I was definitely procrastinating and I needed to do my inventory. I felt spiritually and emotionally broken and I didn't want to feel that way, so I started with my list of resentments, which, if unresolved, can often lead addicts to

44

relapse. We don't have the privilege of holding onto resentments, and I have always found it easy to hold a grudge. There were many people and places I held resentments toward: my first girlfriend, my father, workplaces I was fired from, and the list goes on. There is something therapeutic about putting pen to paper and facing these resentments. When I listed who or what I was angry with and why, I found that harboring these resentments prevented me from freeing my spirit. It was becoming obvious that a life which includes deep resentment leads only to futility and unhappiness.

When someone does something that might hurt my feelings, I sometimes jokingly say to myself, "You just made it into my Fourth Step." For me, making light of something in this way prevents an actual resentment from taking hold. I have always had a good sense of humor, so I use my ability to see the funny side of things to lighten my mood and keep resentment at bay.

I also had to maintain some perspective when I wrote about my sexual relationships. When I was eighteen, my heart was broken, so for the next eleven years I chose not to have a real girlfriend. Girls just got in the way of my using anyway, I told myself. I broke many hearts in the coming years because I still had normal human desires, so I let women believe they were my girlfriends just so they would continue having sex with me. When they found out I was also seeing other women, I would let them go without caring one bit. I look back on this attitude and behavior toward women with great disgrace. The list I made was shamefully extensive and included some women whose names I couldn't even recall.

My inventory also included my deepest, darkest secrets. Resentments and sexual relations were hard, but this was something I really dreaded. I had a couple of things I swore I would take to the grave with me, but these were the things I later found out I most needed to share. I couldn't even write some of them on paper for fear that my writing would

45

somehow be discovered, but I knew I would have to share them in my Fifth Step and I didn't look forward to it.

This concluded my Fourth Step. My sponsor told me that as long as my list was thorough and I got everything out on paper, it would be time for the Fifth Step. The thought of sharing these atrocities with someone else really scared me, but I told myself, "One thing at a time." When I finally made an extensive "searching and fearless moral inventory" of myself, my work on the Fourth Step was completed.

SUDDENLY, I SAW THE TRUTH

Why should I write a list of all my past pain? I had spent years, successfully I thought, putting that pain behind me. I was proud of the fact that I had dealt with and moved beyond my past through years of psychotherapy. Now my sponsor was asking me to dredge up all my past pain. It seemed ridiculous and harmful. But since I had lost my job, was being threatened with lawsuits by multiple people, and had been struggling with depression and suicide for my first six months clean, I figured I didn't have much to lose.

So I wrote…and I wrote…and I wrote…about all the misery in my childhood: my borderline-crazy mom who tormented me, my father who left me with her, the friends who rejected me, the fiancé who abandoned me, the employers who fired me, the boyfriends who used me, and on and on. My sponsor told me to write about those who hurt me, what they did, and how it affected me. I wrote page after page, pouring out years of pain, loneliness, rejection, abandonment, fear, and sorrow. I cried as I wrote each entry. I remembered and felt the pain all over again. I felt my little-girl fears and aches. I felt my big-girl hatred—of "them" and me. I felt ashamed and guilty. My feeling of not being good enough for my mom welled up in my heart again. The feeling of not being good enough for my fiancé hurt me too. I felt like an impostor at work and was terrified of being found out. I found myself slipping into a very negative place. I even began thinking about how pills would take away the emotional pain. I hated writing my Fourth Step.

When I met with my sponsor and started reading my lists to her, she asked me, "So, what's your part in it?" What a stupid question! I had no part in it. My employers didn't see my unique and important contributions to the organization. My mother was mentally ill. My fiancé was selfish and mean. What was my part? Nothing!

But as we worked and talked together about my Fourth Step, she gently introduced my part. Although my mother had been cruel and harmful and I had no responsibility for that as a child, I had carried that pain around for years and had been cruel to her as an adult. My sponsor suggested that my employers might have been turned off by my selfish or defensive attitude. Perhaps my fiancé had left because of my addiction, whether to pills, work, or self-pity.

Suddenly, I saw the truth. I was not a victim, but an active participant in creating my unhappiness. I was shocked! Maybe I really did have a part in much of the misery of my life. And if I had a part in creating it, then I could choose not to create it. I felt empowered, knowing that the world was not a horrible, painful place to live. Perhaps things could be different in the future. I needed to learn a new way of living and interacting with people. But first, I would need to work with God on removing my character defects and then make amends to those I had harmed. Step Four was the beginning of freedom, but much work was still needed.

Working Step Four

Working Step Four can seem like a daunting task. However, as others have found in their recovery, the discovery process is certainly worth the effort. With the help, guidance, and encouragement of our sponsor, we will be able to take stock of our lives, one inventory item at a time. Here are some questions we found helpful to consider and answer in writing before beginning our Fourth Step inventory:

1. Why does my recovery involve more than abstinence from using pills and all other mind-altering substances?

2. What benefits can I expect to see as a result of making a fearless and thorough moral inventory?

3. Why is it important that I not procrastinate about making this inventory, and what are some of the risks of procrastination? What are some of the benefits of *not* procrastinating?

4. How will working with a sponsor and talking and listening to other addicts reassure me that I can handle whatever is revealed in my inventory?

5. How will working this step show my positive qualities, such as honesty, courage, faith, and willingness?

6. Does the word "moral" bother me, and am I afraid I will not be able to live up to society's expectations?

7. How do my current ideas about what is right and wrong compare with society in general? Are there any differences between my own beliefs and society's moral standards?

After answering the above questions, it is time to write out our inventory. Some of us prefer to answer the questions that follow, while others prefer to use a chart format. The choice is ours, but we should discuss both of these methods with our sponsor before deciding which one to use.

In our first Fourth Step, most of us cover our major resentments, fears, sexually related harms, other harms, and assets. As we work on this step, more resentments, fears, harms, or assets may come up and we can certainly add those, but at some point, we must stop and move on. The advice of our sponsor is invaluable in deciding when we have written enough. Since these personal inventories are part of a life-long process by which we keep our house in order, we can always revisit the Fourth Step to add new or newly remembered inventory items, but we cannot use this as an excuse to leave anything out when we work the Fourth Step for the first time.

QUESTION FORMAT

RESENTMENTS

1. What people, institutions, organizations, or beliefs do I resent or have I resented in the past? Describe the situations and circumstances that caused these resentments.

2. What were the motivations or beliefs that caused me to form these resentments and act as I did in these situations?

3. How did I feel threatened in each of these situations?

4. Did I do anything wrong, or have any part in creating the situations that led to these resentments?

5. How does my dishonesty cause me to experience resentments?

6. How does my fear of or my inability to experience certain feelings cause me to develop resentments?

7. How have my resentments influenced my relationships with myself, with other people, or with a Higher Power? How have my resentments cut me off from these relationships and isolated me?

FEAR

1. How have I cheated myself out of positive experiences because of fear?

2. What fears do I have about exposing myself, and about the consequences of doing so?

3. Who, or what, do I fear?

4. How have I been destructive because of these fears? How have I tried to cover up these fears or act as if they did not exist?

FEELINGS

1. How can I identify and understand my feelings? How can I now allow myself to have feelings?

2. Who, or what, can trigger my feelings? What feelings are triggered? What are the situations that present these triggers? Where do my feelings come from (my part)?

3. What were the true motives behind these feelings and how did they cause me to act out in the way that I did?

4. What can I do with my feelings once I have identified them?

GUILT AND SHAME

1. Who, or what, in my life do I have feelings of guilt or shame about? What were the situations and circumstances that led to those feelings?

2. Which of those situations caused me to feel guilt or shame even though I had no part in them?

3. In those situations in which I had a part; what beliefs, feelings, or motivations caused me to act as I did? How have my own actions caused me to have guilt and shame?

RELATIONSHIPS

1. What negative aspects of my personality have made it difficult for me to form friendships or other

relationships? What has made it hard for me to maintain relationships?

2. Have I compulsively looked for superficial relationships?

3. How and why have I avoided intimacy in my relationships?

4. Have I ever ended a relationship for fear of getting hurt?

5. Do I believe my family relationships are stuck in the same patterns, with no hope of change? What is my part in that?

6. Have I felt like a victim in my relationships because of my own unrealistic expectations?

7. Have I considered the feelings and needs of others *and* myself in my relationships? For example, compared to other people, do I consider my feelings more important, less important, or equally important?

8. Did I join clubs or membership organizations only to quit because I felt that my needs were not being met?

9. What are my feelings about work associates, people I went to school with, neighbors, and other similar relationships?

10. Have I ever been institutionalized (treatment center, psychiatric hospital, prison) or held against my will? Did I follow the rules or try to break the rules? How has that affected my personality and attitudes?

11. Have I ever left a relationship rather than work to resolve a conflict?

12. Does my personality change according to the people with whom I associate?

13. What action can I take to change my personality and develop healthy attitudes about relationships?

SEX

1. Have I ever tried to use sex to avoid loneliness or fill a spiritual void, and yet still felt alone and empty?

2. Have I been unable to tell the difference between sex and love? How has acting on that confusion caused me to feel guilt and shame?

3. In what ways was my sexual behavior selfish?

4. How have my sexual practices hurt myself or hurt others?

ABUSE

1. Have I been physically or emotionally abused in the past? Who do I remember abusing me and in what way? When do I remember that abuse occurring? How do I remember feeling after the abuse occurred? What feelings do I still have because of the abuse? Have I continued to feel like a victim because of that abuse?

2. Have I ever abused anyone in any way? Who and how? Was I acting sanely when doing so?

3. What were my feelings after doing so?

4. Did I make excuses, try to justify my actions, or blame my victim? Describe this.

5. What actions can I take, with the help of my Higher Power, to help me be restored to spiritual wholeness?

ASSETS

1. What are some of the things I like about myself?

2. What are some of the things about me that other people like?

3. What are some of my past accomplishments and what hopes do I have for the future?

4. How have my good qualities begun to surface in my recovery? Which of these character assets have grown the most and how?

SECRETS

1. Are there any secrets I have not disclosed in my Fourth Step? What are they?

CHART FORMAT

In this alternative format, we outline our inventory in a chart format. We use as much space as needed in each row to allow us to include sufficient detail about the issue we are addressing. As in the question format, we also begin with a review of resentments.

RESENTMENTS

In this section, we list details in each column:

I am or was resentful at: In this column we list all the people, institutions, and principles we have (or previously had) resentments against.

Because: Under this heading we identify why we have the resentment. What was done to cause the resentment? If there are multiple resentments related to this person, institution, or principle, we list them all.

This affected my: In this column we choose one or more ways that we felt threatened or hurt by each situation listed in the "Because:" column. These may include self-esteem, pride, emotional security, financial security, sexual relationships, personal relationships, and social standing.

What did I do, and why? Here we write about how we responded to each situation and to the person(s) involved in or affected by the circumstances. We also list one or more character defects that were responsible for the actions we have just described. These traits include, but are not limited to: selfishness, dishonesty, fear, lust, vanity, greed, arrogance, perfectionism, anger, conceit, grandiosity, envy, jealousy, distrust, self-pity, laziness, gluttony, intolerance, irresponsibility, procrastination, and lack of consideration.

It might be helpful to use an example to demonstrate the process:

As a teenager I resented my dad because he criticized me and grounded me. This affected my self-esteem and I stayed out all night because I was so angry.

Later on, I developed resentments against my spouse, who always wanted to spend money on things I didn't care about, so I divorced her.

To address these issues, my chart might look like this:

I am or was resentful at:	Because:	This affected my:	What did I do, and why?
Dad	He criticized me and grounded me	Self-esteem	I made him worry by staying out all night: anger, arrogance, lack of consideration
Spouse	Spent money against my wishes	Financial security	Divorced her and refused to pay alimony: greed, anger, and envy.

After completing the Resentments section, we look over our work and add any additional resentments we hold against people, institutions, or principles, now or in the past. Next, we begin the Fears section, completing one column at a time, and then move on to inventory our sexual conduct. We then review any other people or institutions we have harmed, including ourselves.

Finally, we inventory our assets, listing the people and groups we have helped or are now helping, describing the good things we have done and the positive qualities exemplified in each incident.

We list as many of our assets as we can think of, and explain how we have used them in the past, as well as in our recovery today. Some examples are: humility, happiness, trustworthiness, courage, confidence, respectfulness, diligence, enthusiasm, patience, modesty, goodwill, honesty, strength, compassion, empathy, acceptance, kindness, optimism, peacefulness, decency, responsibility, supportiveness, unselfishness, graciousness, hopefulness, forgiveness, restraint, tolerance, fairness, sincerity, openness, fidelity, gratitude, generosity, integrity, faith, willingness, open-mindedness, and serenity.

Here are samples of the charts, one for each section of our inventory. We have only shown two lines for each section to save space, but as many lines as needed should be added to complete the inventory. We also adjust the height and width of each column to accommodate our needs. In actual practice, our writing in the second and fourth columns will generally require the most space.

1. REVIEW OF RESENTMENTS

I am or was resentful at:	Because:	This affected my:	What did I do, and why?

2. Review of Fears

I am or was afraid of:	Because:	This affected my:	What did I do, and why?

3. Review of Sexual Conduct

Who I harmed:	Because:	This affected my:	What did I do, and why?

4. Review of Others We Harmed

Who I harmed:	Because:	This affected my:	What did I do, and why?

5. Listing and Review of Our Assets

Who I helped or benefitted:	What did I do, and why?	Positive traits exhibited:

STEP FIVE

"Admitted to God, to ourselves, and to another human being the exact nature of our wrongs."

Spiritual Principles: Integrity, Truth, Courage

Having completed our inventory in Step Four, we may be feeling quite emotionally raw and vulnerable. If we have been thorough, as Step Four asks us to be, we will have uncovered parts of ourselves that may be difficult to look at. For this reason we will want to do our Fifth Step as soon as possible after completing Step Four. Pills were often the great escape, especially from our negative feelings and self-hatred. Many of us had become adept at running from our problems, ignoring them or hiding in isolation. These familiar behaviors may have a strong pull when we are faced with the realities of our past.

It is natural to feel some fear and anxiety about telling our secrets to another person and God. Self-disclosure exposes us to the possibility of judgment, criticism, and rejection. Feelings of inadequacy and unworthiness have shadowed our lives for many years. Certainly it would be insane to risk exposing our delicate psyches to further damage. We need not worry. If we have been thorough in our work thus far, we will have established the beginnings of a firm foundation. We have come to believe and trust in a power greater than ourselves. We have faith that this power will care for us and have our best interests at heart. We have seen this power at work in our own lives and in the lives of fellow pill addicts in recovery. We listen to the assurance of others and trust that to avoid moving forward with this step would mean missing out on the healing we will experience by releasing ourselves from the bondage of our pasts. The deepest, darkest secrets we have sworn to hold private until death have been like poison to our spirit. Unspoken deeds causing shame and regret have kept us feeling alienated from those around us. Our secrets have blinded us to our better selves. As heard around the rooms of recovery, our secrets keep us sick.

We cannot afford to take this step on our own or insanity will return; and eventually, we will use again. Left to our own thinking and judgment, it is easy for us to rationalize and minimize our actions when looking at our pasts. We can also be very good at self-condemnation and overly exaggerating our faults. When we tell our story to another person, he or she provides us with a more balanced perspective. There are details of our lives that we have never shared with another human being. These secrets have festered in the darkness of our fear, shame, and self-hatred. When we bring our secrets into the light by sharing them with someone we trust, we feel a great sense of release and freedom.

Often, the person with whom we share will tell us parts of his or her story. We suddenly feel a strong, compassionate connection with another human being and we know deep down that we are not alone in the world.

Most of us have taken this step with our sponsor. Having had his or her help walking through the first four steps, we often find that doing Step Five with our sponsor strengthens our relationship even further. Our relationship with our sponsor will likely take on a deeper significance upon completing Step Five. Sharing our Fifth Step with another recovering addict allows the opportunity for an exchange of emotions that only those who have walked in the shoes of active addiction can know. We find ourselves sharing tears and laughter for our common struggles and our absurd attempts to maintain our unmanageable lives. It can actually feel good to let it out! However, some addicts do not share their Fifth Step with their sponsor, choosing instead a spiritual advisor or someone else they trust. It is important that the person we select understand what a Fifth Step is. He or she should be a person of integrity who will keep our story in confidence, someone who will respect our feelings, and focus on keeping us on track as to the exact nature of our wrongs or shortcomings when we confuse our part with another's. Remember, our purpose is to clean our house.

We may think that admitting to God the exact nature of our wrongs is a bit silly. God should already know these things, right? In becoming honest with the God of our understanding we take this spiritual relationship to a deeper level. Step Five assists us in continuing to clear the way for the bright light of our spirit to shine in our lives. In Steps Two and Three we asked for, and started to develop, the spiritual principles of trust and faith. Now we turn to this power greater than ourselves and ask for courage: the courage to speak the truth, the courage to be honest about ourselves and about our past with another human being, and the courage to acknowledge and accept the nature of our wrongs. Alone or with our sponsor, we can ask the God of our understanding to be present as we tell our story, asking for the grace to help us be thorough. Formally inviting this power greater than ourselves into our Fifth Step—through a simple prayer—can only serve to expand our relationship with the God of our understanding.

As we grow in our recovery, we may find the need to revisit Step Five. As our minds and bodies heal from the disease of addiction, we will naturally experience greater clarity about our past and present circumstances. We learn that feelings of uneasiness and fear are cues for us to open up to our sponsor about unfinished business or current struggles. We remember to be searching and fearless, whether we are facing our first Fifth Step or working this step again, years into our recovery.

Upon completion of this step, we find we have been granted the courage we asked for, and more. We feel accepted, character defects and all. Our sense of isolation is replaced with a feeling of belonging. Perhaps for the first time we have a profound experience of feeling a part of and connected. We begin to know humility; we are teachable. We are not 'better than' or 'less than'; we simply see who we truly are. Having released the weight of the heavy baggage of our past, it is quite natural that we will feel the incredible lightness of self-acceptance and serenity. Fears fall away and leave room for the spirit of peace. All of this, wrapped together in grace, is evidence of a deepening God-consciousness. With this awareness and energy, we move on to Step Six.

OUR MEMBERS' EXPERIENCE WITH STEP FIVE

GOD'S FLASHLIGHT

At the age of thirty-five, I crawled through the doors of a treatment center, broken and dying. How in the world had this happened? I had been using drugs and alcohol recreationally since I was fifteen, but, my recent five-year love affair with pain pills had brought me to my knees. This was not a typical love affair. I had desperately wanted to end this abusive relationship for years, but could not. During the first days of my love affair with pills, the euphoria fulfilled what I thought to be my wildest dreams! When we were "together," I was magnificent, beautiful, powerful, confident, wickedly smart, and invincible. I was filled with (what I thought was) a great love for everyone around me. I was completely numb to physical or emotional pain. I believed I could and would conquer the world! I considered myself to have been nothing and no one before pills. This was the love I had been searching for my whole life. Finally, I was complete. But all great things come to an end.

Months into our relationship, I began to have a vague feeling that things weren't quite right. It began as a distant, impending sense of doom during our times of brief separation. I wanted the pills all the time. I used more and more for the same effect. I tried to control the amount I used, with no luck. My need progressed into unimaginably severe physical withdrawals and emotional agony until we were reunited. I came to need the pills all the time just to feel normal. Without them, I was sick, ugly, stupid, lazy, worthless, angry, bitter, and resentful. I hated myself and the world around me. By the time I realized I needed to put an end to the madness and quit the relationship, it was too late. I wanted to stop, but my willpower was nonexistent. I had become a full-blown addict. My crazy-train had left the station and I was powerless to get off, no matter what.

Years passed as my abuse continued and the consequences mounted. I used the relationship I had with my pills to live, and lived to use more pills. My former self was unrecognizable. I was insane and delusional. I was self-centered and paranoid. I couldn't look anyone in the eye, nor could I remember the last time I had laughed or even cracked a smile. I lost my moral compass: I lied, manipulated, and committed fraud to keep this abuser in my life. I stopped speaking with my family and friends. I dropped out of medical school. I couldn't hold down a job and I was deeply in debt. I stopped eating and I looked skeletal. My body was so deteriorated that I could no longer have children. I was going to die and I prayed for death every day…but God had other plans.

The sixty-day stint in a treatment center saved my life. After about five weeks of physical detoxification, the fog cleared and I began to learn a few things. This was my first introduction to the Twelve Steps. First, I learned I wasn't the only one stuck in the insane loop of powerlessness and unmanageability. Unbeknownst to me, I had been having a Step One experience for years. I began to understand that the First Step implies that I was going to use pills no matter what, and that I was completely powerless to stop. In addition, I learned that I had been in this state of perpetual delusion, thinking I had the power to control my using. My counselor used an analogy to describe my delusion of control: "You jumped off the roof of a building and halfway down you thought, 'I think I'll hit the pavement!'" He also told me that I'd been changed from a cucumber to a pickle, and that there was no turning back: "Once an addict, always an addict," he told me.

I learned that hope came in with Steps Two and Three. I came to believe and made a decision to allow a power greater than myself to return me to sanity. It didn't matter how I defined that power (Universal Harmony, Creator, Spirit of the Universe, Nature, God, whatever), as long as it was a power *greater than myself* and it wasn't my own ego or thinking. For hadn't my own best thinking gotten me into rehab? At the time, I wasn't really sure if this power would work, but I was at least willing to believe it was possible. Apparently, that was all that was needed.

Even though the drugs were out of my system for five weeks and my physical cravings were gone, I was experiencing constant, full-blown mental obsessions to get loaded. I felt like I was coming out of my skin! I learned mental obsessions come in many forms: thoughts of using, thoughts of not using, resentments, etc. Intense fear was driving my every selfish thought and self-seeking action. I was desperately searching for approval from others, acting obnoxious, blaming others for how I felt, gossiping, and feeling a deep sense of self-pity, bitterness, and anger. I was a total train wreck. This is what some say is "white-knuckled" clean time. Not fun.

This led me to my Fourth Step. My sponsor gave me my Step Four assignment. I was told if I didn't do my Fourth Step inventory soon, I was doomed to get loaded again. I believed it! I wasn't going to be able to carry around all this anger and fear for much longer. I needed to get down on paper all of the fears and resentments I'd been carrying around since the time I could remember. Who did I resent, why, and where was I at fault? The last part would be tricky. I believed I wasn't at fault with any of it, and I was certain my sponsor would agree with me!

The amazing thing about my sponsor was that she smacked me out of my delusional thinking—it was almost as if she hit me on the head with a two-by-four. We met for my Fifth Step. I read her all the resentments and fears I'd written about in my Fourth Step. My sponsor helped me see my part and take total responsibility for my actions over the years. I was astounded at the notion that all of my problems were of my own making! In fact, I was given a long list of character defects that I could call my own: selfishness, manipulation, victimization, blaming, dishonesty, self-righteousness, controlling, and people-pleasing, just to name a few. Some of my core fears included the fear of not being good enough, being unlovable, unworthy, rejected, disliked, and judged. I had been using these defects and fears to navigate through my entire life.

This very first Fifth Step (I've done more than a few since then) was the most freeing experience of my life! Knowing I was the problem meant I could also be the solution! I felt so incredibly empowered. Steps Six and Seven involved my being ready and willing to have God remove those things about my personality that had made me useless to myself and those around me. That night I prayed, asking God to remove my resentments, defects, and fears. Within two days, I stopped having mental obsessions about pills. I no longer felt anger toward those I had included in my Fourth Step. It was an absolute miracle! I felt lighter, more buoyant. It was as if God shined a flashlight into my brain and everything became illuminated. I was awake, aware, and conscious.

The Fifth Step was the turning point for me in my recovery. Once God helped me remove all that garbage from my mind and soul, I was free to complete the rest of the steps, be of service, and guide other suffering addicts through their recovery journeys. Pills Anonymous became my home, and my best friends in the world are members of the P.A. Fellowship. That shell of a person that I was years ago is no longer. She is gone and I have been reborn.

NOTHING LEFT TO HIDE

Because of Step Five and a lot of hard work and honesty with myself and my sponsor, I am at peace with my past. This step really helped me see the person I became as a result of my pill addiction. Looking back now, I can see how far I have come, and that is an amazing feeling I carry with me in my heart.

Just thinking about the Fifth Step caused anxiety for me, but I knew if I wanted to get better I had to do it. When I began to write my inventory, I felt overwhelmed by the things I had done. To even think about breathing my deepest, darkest secrets to another human being made me want to run away— but I didn't, and pushed on.

I put a piece of paper on my counter and wrote down the first few thoughts that had been weighing on my heart the most. Then, as the days passed, I jotted down a few more thoughts when I had time. As I got more honest with myself, more was being revealed.

Before I went to meet with my sponsor, I read over what I had written a few times to make sure I hadn't left out anything. That paper in my hand was full of my baggage. Just having it all down in writing scared me, but it also gave less power to the guilt I had carried with me for years like a heavy backpack weighing me down.

As I spilled my guts to my sponsor, I couldn't believe how many times she said, "Me, too!" or, "That's not so bad." She didn't even blink an eye when I told her about all the people I had intentionally or unintentionally hurt. After I finished, we walked away from that table closer friends. I immediately asked if I could throw away the paper or burn it. My sponsor laughed and left it up to me.

This was the first time I felt that the program could really help me forgive myself and move on from the person I used to be. The wreckage I had created in my life was starting to feel less poisonous. The next day I felt lighthearted, like a huge weight had been lifted from me. For the first time I felt like I didn't have anything to hide. I couldn't believe how something as simple as sharing the past could affect my present and, in turn, my future as well

This was my favorite step for one main reason. When I worked the Fifth Step with my sponsor, I could literally *feel* the difference from one day to the next. And, of course, as an addict I loved the instant gratification. Taking pills used to be all that I looked forward to. I counted them in the morning to see how many I had left. I worked all day connecting with the people who could get me more. It really consumed my life. Now I live a simple life, growing slowly each day, and making efforts to become the person I have always wanted to be.

WORKING STEP FIVE

As we approached this step, many of us felt relief at the completion of Step Four, but we felt apprehensive about sharing our faults and secrets with anyone else. Answering these questions, with the guidance of a sponsor that we have come to know and trust, can help us find the courage to admit the exact nature of our wrongs to God, ourselves, and another human being.

1. What are my hopes and fears about sharing my faults and secrets with someone else?

2. What is it about the person who will hear my Fifth Step that I connect with, that makes me feel comfortable about making my admissions? What are the specific qualities that make him (or her) the right person to hear my Fifth Step? (For instance: trustworthiness, commitment to recovery, being non-judgmental, and having a positive attitude.)

3. Am I willing to turn my will over to my Higher Power and trust the person who will hear my Fifth Step?

4. What are my expectations about the person who will listen to my Fifth Step?

5. How will I develop a new understanding about how to participate in relationships as a result of working Step Five?

6. Why is it important to discuss and understand the exact nature of my wrongs and not just the wrong actions themselves? What is the difference between my wrong actions and the exact nature of my wrongs?

7. How have I practiced self-deception while avoiding self-honesty in the past, and how does working Step Five help me come to accept myself?

OUR MEMBERS' EXPERIENCE
WITH STEP SIX

RECOGNIZING THE PAY-OFF

The very first time I read Step Six, I quickly surmised that there wasn't much to it and wondered why they even included it with the other eleven steps. Having adopted a troubleshooting method of putting out fires in my chaotic life, Step Six didn't appear to have much substance to it. There were no lists to create and check off, and no direct actions that some of the other steps suggested.

Entirely ready? Of course I was. The reality of my personality defects was slowly starting to sink in after taking an inventory in Step Five. Sharing this inventory with my sponsor was initially a relief, but I was soon dismayed at the realization that I wasn't who I thought I was. Being medicated on pills, I never thought of myself as an angry or depressed person, except when I tried to quit. However, with some clean time behind me, the message was clear—that my personality more closely resembled that of a child than an adult. And it was also evident that other people I associated with—fellow employees, neighbors, people I attend meetings with, and family members—most likely see me as I really am.

Yes, I was ready to have God remove this defective personality, full of resentment, jealousy, envy, fear, depression, self-pity, and the other entirely negative by-products of false pride such as gossip, name-dropping, and sarcasm. So I bypassed Step Six and formally asked God to remove these character defects as we are guided in Step Seven. Confident that I was going to be transformed into a spiritual wonder, I went forward with high hopes that I would be free of this personality at last. But I soon found out that my shortcomings were not going away, even after repeated requests in prayer. I would start off each day asking God to remove specific defects that were causing the most problems. Anger directed toward people who didn't act the way I thought they should was my most glaring and repetitive personality defect. Gossiping at work was another. And fear of the future headed the list.

So when my repeated efforts failed, I called my sponsor about my predicament. He reminded me of my work in the Fourth and Fifth Steps and the importance of understanding the exact nature of my wrongs. And he also guided me back to the Sixth Step, which focuses on willingness and readiness, not on asking for our defects to be removed.

He asked me to write down what the payoff was for gossip, anger, and fear. Gossip was easy to see. There was kind of an excitement or rush when gossiping about another employee at work, especially if I felt bored. I never felt good about myself afterwards but it seemed automatic, like I was unconscious when doing it. My sponsor pointed out that gossip gave him a temporary feeling of superiority by pointing out some negative aspect of another person. I had to admit to myself that I felt the same way.

It was a bit more difficult to see any short-term payoff from anger. My sponsor explained to me that, just like gossip, anger at the misbehavior or character defects of others was a way of temporarily feeling superior to them. He also disclosed that he was usually annoyed by people whose personalities were similar to his. This was difficult to see, but after careful examination, I realized that people who struck me as being self-centered bigmouths bothered me the most, and I had to painfully admit that I matched that profile.

When I thought about the benefit I was deriving from being in constant fear of the future, I was puzzled. Again, I sought my sponsor's help. He shared his own experience that early in his recovery he was also in constant fear. He said his fear was so great that he was often paralyzed to take action for fear that he might make the wrong decision. He discovered that when he stayed in fear, he felt justified in putting off decisions, but the underlying motive was his fear of making the wrong decisions and failing. He worried, "What would people think of me if I failed?" This made sense to me when I looked back at my life and saw all of my own inaction and avoidance. I thought I was lazy, but the actual driving force was my self-centered interest in protecting my image so I could look good.

Although I thought I was entirely ready to have God remove my defects of character, I needed the Sixth Step to learn that I was receiving short-term benefits in the form of ego boosts. It was only through this painful admission of the "exact nature of my wrongs" that I was really ready to have God remove my shortcomings in Step Seven.

THE WILLINGNESS TO BE WILLING

I learned in Steps Four and Five that my character defects were the reason I had been angry, restless, irritable, and discontented. I thought I was entirely ready to have God remove these defects. However, no matter how unhealthy the reasons, these traits had served a purpose in my life.

As a result of the trauma and abuse I experienced in my early childhood, I had built a wall around myself. My jealousy, arrogance, anger, blaming of others, self-justification, self-pity, self-victimization, unwillingness to forgive, and being excessively judgmental helped me to keep the wall up, and to keep everyone at arm's length. These attitudes were unhealthy coping mechanisms that I acquired from an early age and continued to build upon throughout my life. My character defects were so embedded and ingrained in my way of thinking that I honestly was not aware they existed until I did my Fifth Step with my sponsor. I always blamed my problems and misery on other people and events in my life. With the help of my sponsor, I learned that these warped attitudes and behaviors were the reason I was miserable and in despair, with absolutely no hope.

As much as I wanted them gone, my defects had been the driving forces in my life. I didn't know how to live without them. Because I did not know how to live without the anger and fear, I had to become willing to learn a new way of living. This was very frightening to consider, and until I was ready to take the risk of change and walk through my fears, I was not willing to let go of these defects. The beauty of Step Six is that I only had to become willing to ask God to remove my shortcomings, so I prayed for the willingness to be willing. Once the willingness came, I was then able to move on to Step Seven and ask God to remove my shortcomings.

The willingness to let go of my defects didn't happen all at once. I was willing to be rid of some more than others. To my surprise, the first defects I became willing to release were anger and blame. But other defects like jealousy and self-pity took longer. It took me quite a while to learn to be happy for other people, to realize that their success didn't take anything away from me. I had always been threatened by others' success because I was so concerned about my own, so instead of being happy when good things happened to people around me, I was jealous and bitter. With time I became willing to work through the real issues behind my jealousy, and became ready to ask God to remove this weakness from my character.

Self-pity kept me in the victim role. My warped way of thinking had consisted of, "Poor me; if you had my life, you would use drugs too." This program has taught me that as a victim, I allow everyone else to determine the course of my life. The willingness to be accountable for my actions and take responsibility for my life was a huge step for me. This meant that I could stop running in circles and begin to take steps forward.

Getting clean didn't make everything in life beautiful and positive. Life still happens and I am still human. Sometimes these defects still raise their ugly heads, but I am now aware of them and immediately ask God to remove them if it is His will. The program of Pills Anonymous has taught me new coping mechanisms and how to live life on life's terms, not my own.

WORKING STEP SIX

In Step Six we categorize and list the character defects that led us to cause the harms we enumerated in Step Four and admitted in Step Five. Making this list is in itself an expression of our readiness to have God remove these defects. We have also discovered that the emotionally exhausting and humbling experience of thoroughly working Step Five can certainly leave us willing, open, and entirely ready to have God remove our defects. However, we must prepare ourselves in other ways. The following questions can lead us to an understanding of our defects and how to go about having them removed.

1. In the process of working my Fourth and Fifth Steps, how aware did I become of my negative character traits?

2. Which of my character defects stand out the most?

3. Which character defects were like survival skills, and how do I feel they protected me when I felt threatened?

4. How did my pill addiction help me to nurture these defects and act out on them?

5. When I acted out on each defect, what effect did it have on me, and on others?

6. What feelings can I match to each defect? Was I trying to hide from or suppress these feelings by my actions?

7. What would my life be like if I could apply or substitute spiritual principles for these defects?

8. Do I have fears about the person I would become as the result of asking God to remove these defects of character? For instance, do I fear that I would not be able to protect myself?

9. What would my life be like today without each of these defects? What specific goals could I attain if I did not have these defects? What opportunities could I recognize and take advantage of, if I did not have these defects? In what ways could I be a better parent, child, friend, spouse, worker, etc. without these defects?

10. How does the quality and resolve of my surrender deepen in this step, and what actions can I take to feel and show that I am entirely ready for God to remove these defects of character?

STEP SEVEN

"Humbly asked Him to remove our shortcomings."

Spiritual Principles: Humility, Trust, Patience

We take our willingness to let go of character defects in Step Six, and shift our focus to the principle of humility in Step Seven by asking God to remove the shortcomings. Once again, we are faced with the fact that we cannot move through life on our own power in order to find peace and release from suffering. Humility means having a modest opinion of one's own importance. Our first encounter with true humility may have been with the First Step when we admitted our powerlessness over pills and all other mind-altering substances. We finally began to surrender in our long, hard-fought battle with control and our own self-will when we were awakened by the dawning revelation that we may not have been the ruler we thought we were. We were not left without a solution, however, as we went on to Steps Two and Three and began our journey with a power greater than ourselves. We found we no longer had to go it alone. When we turned our will and our lives over to the care of the God of our understanding, this power was available to work in our lives. This relationship of faith and trust aids us again and again as we work our program of recovery.

We gained insight by honestly looking at our shortcomings. Seeing how we lived our lives under the control of our character defects has given us fresh perspective. Our new awareness has given us a willingness to let go of those parts of ourselves that caused us—and continue to cause us—despair, frustration, bewilderment, fear, loneliness, and suffering. We now want freedom from anything that limits our recovery. Like trying to control our use of pills in the end, we find that on our own, we have no power to remove these shortcomings despite our good intentions. Step Seven takes us back into surrender. We have discovered much about ourselves in our work thus far. Our defects may have made us miserable, but we are no longer blind. We accept ourselves and we are now willing to take responsibility for our lives. We take a step further in our relationship with God in another act of trust as we humbly ask our Higher Power for help.

Step Seven moves us farther from self-reliance and closer to God-reliance. Many of us came into recovery in a state of spiritual bankruptcy. We had no concept of spirituality. We only felt a deep hole in the center of our being that could not be filled no matter how hard we tried. We were stranded on a raft of desperation with no direction, dying as we tried to fill that spiritual void with pills. As long as we lived our lives on self-propulsion and total self-reliance, we blocked the full potential for the sunshine of the spirit to pour into our lives. Through working the Twelve Steps with a sponsor, going to meetings, and talking to other recovering pill addicts, we begin to feel that hole being filled—sometimes quickly, sometimes slowly, but filled nonetheless. That desperate grasping and clinging for things that fed our defects is replaced with a new sense of direction. No longer is there a deep ache and hunger that cannot be satisfied. We are being filled with a spirit of love, forgiveness, and gratitude as we learn to live our lives according to spiritual principles. The people in our lives have been observing this transformation since we began working our program of recovery. At times we may have experienced frustration, fear, anger, and doubt over our progress, but with every effort, every step, we have been changing slowly, but surely. As we experience this deepening awakening of our spirit, we realize with certainty that we are no longer the same broken, hopeless people who walked into Pills Anonymous for the first time.

Working Step Seven requires not only humility, but also patience. Shortcomings are like weeds. They keep popping up. We are asking for help to change a lifetime of conditioning. Awareness, perseverance, and acceptance of our humanness are important here. We are not saints. We do not strive to be perfect human beings. We remain mindful of our expectations. Step Seven can be taken as often as we need. We may ask for a "blanket" removal of our shortcomings on a daily basis, or pray for a particular trait to be removed when the occasion warrants. As our shortcomings present themselves, we turn to our Higher Power.

Prayer is simply communication with our Higher Power and can take any form. The more we practice communication with our Higher Power, the more we are reassured by the serenity we experience when we pray. When turning to our Higher Power in Step Seven, we may say a simple prayer such as:

> God, I open myself to the power of Your love. Please take away those parts of my character that no longer serve You or others. Use me as a channel of Your peace as I walk in recovery.

It is possible to experience immediate release, but removal of our shortcomings is usually a progressive washing away. In any case, with adherence to this practice of communicating with our Higher Power, we will find ourselves experiencing relief. This does not mean that we will not encounter the consequences of our character defects again, for this is a lifetime journey. It does mean that through awareness, prayer, and change, we will find a new and more peaceful path in life and in recovery. As we see results, our faith and trust in our Higher Power will grow. We are becoming more comfortable with edging our egos out, and allowing God's power in.

As with the first six steps, we ask our sponsor to help guide us through Step Seven. We are fortunate to benefit from his or her experience, strength, and hope as we move forward in recovery. Having the assistance of another addict is a tremendous blessing for us and represents another opportunity to open ourselves to the spiritual principle of humility. We strive to remain teachable throughout our recovery journey.

We have defined new objectives for ourselves since we came to Pills Anonymous and began actively working our recovery. We find we enjoy fellowship and getting along with others. The peace we experience as a result of our efforts has become a valued commodity. The resulting serenity we experience from doing the next right thing is a powerful motivator to stay the course when shortcomings threaten to push us over the edge into past behavioral patterns. We have acquired many tools to assist us in living a life with which we can feel comfortable. Our efforts and the spiritual muscle we have gained have prepared us for the work we have yet to do in Step Eight. We move forward with a spirit of courage, faith, and perseverance.

OUR MEMBERS' EXPERIENCE WITH STEP SEVEN

MR. PERFECTIONIST

When I reached Step Seven, it was the same as when I reached all the other steps. The work I had done on the previous steps prepared me to do the work necessary for the next step. I had seemingly surrendered in Step One. I resigned as general manager of the universe in Steps Two and Three. I purged my soul and became accountable in Steps Four and Five, and I decided I was ready for this new way of life in Step Six. But now, the Seventh Step was asking me to be willing to give it all over to a power in the universe greater than myself, and was suggesting that I exhibit humility.

Me: Mr. Perfectionist, Mr. Impatient, Mr. Always-Have-To-Be-In-Control! I had to face all these character defects, realize they had never served me well, and become willing to ask for help to be rid of them.

Taking pills was not just about pain relief for me. At the outset it was, but over time, using pills was also about numbing emotions. If I did not feel emotion, then I did not have to think about how miserable I thought my life was. The pills allowed me to go on and not have to be Mr. Anything.

When I worked Step Seven, I finally realized that I could not handle life alone—and I couldn't manage life with pills either. I came to understand that I did not have to go it alone anymore. The God of my understanding would help me, would never abandon me, and would show me the path He had laid out for me in His own good time. All I had to do was set aside my ego and humbly ask for help. If I did that, then I could continue progressing through the steps to a life far more spectacular than I could ever imagine.

The Seventh Step was the "climb-the-mountain" step for me. It was the "real" surrender step for me. If I would just cloak myself in God, humbly ask for His guidance and help, and climb each step up that mountain by practicing the new ways of thinking and behaving I had been shown, then I would be able to leave my old ways behind.

I am grateful I was beaten into submission by my pill addiction because the humility I came to know in my heart allowed me to work this step. For me, humility means subduing my independence, power, and will. What a tremendous relief to know that I do not have to be completely self-sufficient anymore, that I do not have to exert my power over others anymore, and that my will can only poison me.

Today, I seek daily interdependence with God. I ask Him to exert His influence over me and help me rid myself of my character defects. In my Seventh Step prayer, I asked God to remove the character defects that stand in the way of my being useful to Him and to others, and to grant me the strength to do so, because I simply do not have the strength to do it alone.

The most powerful realization of Step Seven was that I never have to be alone or face any travail in life by myself. God wants me to be happy! By accepting the good that comes from deflating my overblown ego, I now fully understand what living a life of recovery means, and this motivates me to stay on the path. I lost so much during my active pill addiction, but I refuse to give back all that I have gained in recovery.

IT'S A PROCESS

The day I entered rehab, I was a scared and lonely pill addict. I had no idea how I was going to stay clean, but I knew that if I was going to stay alive any longer, I had to be willing to do whatever they told me to do. It seemed very simple. Go to meetings, get a sponsor, and work the steps. One thing I knew for sure was that I had really messed up my life trying to do it my way, and I had to try another way.

I found Pills Anonymous shortly after spending thirty days in rehab. I had bounced around a couple of other fellowships, trying different meetings, but I was a pill addict. I knew that I was "home" just a few minutes into my first P.A. meeting. Soon I found a sponsor, and started working the steps. I had tackled Step One in rehab and in therapy, and I worked it a third time with my sponsor. One of my friends in recovery told me that it's the only step we have to do perfectly, and I became pretty good at it.

I moved on, spending a long time on Steps Four and Five for the usual reasons, and then moved on to Step Six. Believe me, I was entirely ready to have God remove my character defects. That part was easy. But then I became quite stuck on Step Seven. My sponsor told me to pray, so pray I did. Ever since I worked Step Two, I had been struggling to find and connect with a power greater than myself. I knew I needed one, because without my Higher Power, I had nowhere to turn.

For years, pills were my Higher Power. I put them before my wife and children, before my friends and family, and before my money and my business. I knew that pills were killing me, but I wanted to live. I realize now that my Higher Power was looking out for me and had plans for my life, but being the addict I am, it took a while for me to learn this.

So I prayed. I asked my Higher Power to remove my shortcomings. I asked and I prayed, and I asked and I prayed again and again, but it seemed that every morning I woke up with the same shortcomings. I felt okay, and things were going well with my recovery and my family, but why wasn't my Higher Power removing my shortcomings? I thought I must not be praying properly or hard enough. It just didn't seem to be working and no one really had any advice other than to keep praying.

Then one day, sitting in a Pills Anonymous meeting, I realized that, like everything in my recovery, it's a process. And then I had another realization. I understood that when I was sitting in a meeting, my failings were not being completely removed, but were being gradually diminished. Suddenly, I felt that the weight of my transgressions was a bit lighter. Wow! And then I had another epiphany. When I'm sitting in a Pills Anonymous meeting, listening to someone share, or sharing myself, my conscious contact with my Higher Power is at its greatest. I realized that Step Seven, like my recovery, is a work in progress. I am so grateful for this program and the things that it teaches me about how to live.

WORKING STEP SEVEN

By working the previous steps we have been doing the spiritual preparation necessary to work Step Seven. Not only have we begun to discover the difference between humiliation and humility, we have also been building a more positive self-image and practicing spiritual principles. We have come to understand the harm we inflicted because of our character defects. We are now ready to ask God to remove our propensity to let our shortcomings rule our lives. Writing out answers to the following questions and discussing them with our sponsor may help us to understand this further.

1. What would my life be like if my Higher Power were to remove even a few of my worst shortcomings?

2. How does the principle of humility affect the process of my recovery? How does my awareness of my own humility help me to work Step Seven?

3. What can get in the way of asking for help (for example: apathy, low self-esteem, ego, and fear)?

4. How can I benefit from listening to other pill addicts share about asking their Higher Power to remove their shortcomings? How can other addicts and my sponsor help me in doing this for myself?

5. Have there been times when I have been able to refrain from acting on a specific character defect and practice a spiritual principle instead? Do I recognize this as God working in my life?

6. How does getting out of the way so my Higher Power can work in my life help me to practice spiritual principles?

7. What action can I take when I become impatient and feel that my shortcomings have not been removed immediately, or as quickly as I asked? Will this action help me be confident that they will eventually be removed, in God's time?

8. How has recovery meant not only exposing shortcomings that need to be eliminated, but also discovering assets that need to be emphasized?

9. What assets would emerge if God removed the character defects I discovered in Steps Four and Five and listed in Step Six?

10. How strongly do I believe that recovery is an ongoing process, and that it is necessary for me to work Step Seven on a continual basis?

STEP EIGHT

"Made a list of all persons we had harmed and became willing to make amends to them all."

Spiritual Principles: Willingness, Honesty, Courage

We continue our spiritual housecleaning in Step Eight. We have looked at our thoughts, our feelings, our actions, and our lives. We have probed deeply to uncover any and all behaviors and character traits that hold us back in our recovery. We have made a thorough examination of ourselves, past and present. As we continue to grow in recovery, our world is becoming bigger. It is no longer just a "me" world. Self-centeredness is slipping away and we are ready to take an important step in healing the damage of our pasts. Shame and guilt may still weigh heavy in our minds and on our hearts. We must be willing to move forward if we are to experience freedom from these burdens. We have been practicing the spiritual principles of honesty, courage, and willingness in our work thus far. We continue to rely on these principles when working Step Eight.

Step Eight asks us to be accountable for our actions by taking responsibility for the harm we caused others. We take responsibility through the process of making amends. To amend is to change, repair, correct, right, or remedy. We resist the temptation to fall into self-righteousness. We do not focus on what others may have done to us in the past. Here, we are concerned with repairing the damage *we* have done. When we look at our past behavior, we cannot avoid responsibility by saying our wrongs were justified by another person's actions. There are no "justifiable wrongs" we inflicted on others. If we hold onto the idea that we somehow justifiably harmed others, we will not do our amends properly and we will remain resentful, which could trigger a relapse.

We ask our Higher Power for the willingness to see the truth of our past behavior. We ask for release from fear and false pride as we look back as far as we are able. Our recovery is a journey. Our Eighth Step list is a living list; it changes and grows over time. As we become ready to see our past, and as we gain more clarity through staying clean and working the Steps, we often find ourselves remembering persons to add to our list. If we get stuck, we ask for the willingness to be willing to make amends. We remember our work in Steps Six and Seven letting go of our character defects. We use the same strategy when wrestling with our thoughts and fears while working Step Eight. Many of us said to our sponsor, "I will never make amends to *that* person! *I* did not hurt them; they harmed *me!*" At times like these, we use the three spiritual principles of Step Eight: willingness, honesty, and courage. If we are simply *willing* to *honestly* consider the possibility that we may have played a part—however small—in whatever occurred, then we will gain the *courage* needed to accept the fact that we owe an amends. Our sponsors can be of great help in these matters because they likely had the same thoughts and feelings, yet with the help of their own sponsors, they were able to break through the fear and continue to move through the Steps. For example, sometimes our sponsor can help us to see that while someone else may have initially caused some harm, our reaction to it may have compounded the problem or made it worse. And if there is still someone with whom we cannot immediately come to terms, we say "not yet," instead of "never." This is the type of honesty we need in order to stay alive. It may not be easy at first to see the wisdom of making amends. We often hear, "It is in the past. Let it be." or "Why open up old wounds?" We must understand that this is the type of thinking that kept us sick and afraid, and in many cases almost killed us. As our trust and spirituality deepen, we are presented with opportunities to make amends, and are moved by a power greater than ourselves to do what we previously could not have done. As we stay the course in recovery, we remain open to the possibility of healing and growth whenever and wherever it may manifest.

Our list will include people, institutions, businesses, organizations, and communities. Reviewing our list from Step Four may help provide us with ideas for names to include on our list. Harm may have involved physical injury, emotional trauma, mental abuse, or spiritual damage. The harm we have done to others may be subtle. Have we acted in ways that aroused anger, jealousy, or fear in others? Have we been irritable, critical, or cold toward others? Have we been so full of self-pity, fear, or depression that we affected those around us? Have we dominated or manipulated those around us? Are we also guilty of "sins of omission"? Have we caused others harm because we were too intoxicated or too self-absorbed to help them when they needed help? The list is endless. We look at the ways in which our character defects— our survival instincts in the extreme—have harmed people in our home, at our workplace, and in our community. Our intentions do not matter. We look at our actions and decide whether we have caused harm. We must be honest about the effects of our actions. Though we may not have intended to do harm, thinking we were only affecting ourselves, this was not always the case. Working Step Eight with a sponsor will help us discriminate between what we thought we were doing and what the result was for those around us. A sponsor will also help us avoid being overly judgmental of ourselves and others.

One very important addition to our list is our own name. On the path of our active addiction, we did great harm to ourselves. We have definitely earned a place on the list and we deserve forgiveness. We come to know what it feels like to stand on both sides of the Eighth Step.

There may be those who belong on our list who we feel have done more harm to us than we have done to them. Again, we pray for the spirit of willingness. We also ask for the spirit of forgiveness. The spiritual principles of willingness and forgiveness will deepen our understanding of humility, and humility will also assist us when making our amends in Step Nine.

We may not be able to approach some of those on our list, or it may prove inappropriate to do so. This should not stop us from including them. We have an opportunity to make what we call "living amends" every day we awake clean. We do this by working our program of recovery to the best of our ability. We stay clean, go to meetings, meet with our sponsor, and talk to and work with other pill addicts. We continue to grow by changing the things we can: the thinking and behaviors that brought us down in the past.

We are careful when doing Step Eight to not fall into morbid self-reflection. The purpose of Step Eight is not to make a list of all those we have harmed so that we feel badly about ourselves. The purpose is to see the truth of how our addiction affected those around us and to take responsibility for those actions. We will then complete the release of our past through Step Nine when we make amends and feel the freedom of making peace with our past. As we take this step, we remember that we also have done good deeds in the past.

We are human, which means that we have lived our life doing the best we could with what we had. We have harmed some and we have helped some. We focus on cleaning up our past so that we can start our new, clean lives free from the negative energy of harms caused by our past behavior.

As a result of our work on Step Eight, we will begin to experience the freedom that comes from feeling closer to others. Our feelings of isolation will begin to dissolve as we feel a renewed connectedness with the world.

OUR MEMBERS' EXPERIENCE
WITH STEP EIGHT

MAKING A LIST, CHECKING IT TWICE

I entered recovery by way of a legal and professional intervention. After sharing my story in a meeting one night, the man who would later be my sponsor said, "Well you really made a name for yourself. How does it feel to be famous, or should I say infamous?" Of course, I felt like I had a target on my back. Only recently, after talking with the DEA agent who spearheaded my intervention, did I learn that the only reason I was allowed to enter a detoxification facility and then rehab instead of incarceration, was that nobody wanted me to die on their watch.

Upon leaving treatment, the amends at the top of my list were federal employees, professionals, and the IRS (I had a couple of "disagreements" with them). I discovered that good news never came by certified mail. These were not discretionary amends. I felt as if I was in a tiny little box. I was being watched, investigated, and tested by two different monitoring programs. If I was to salvage a twenty-year career, stay out of another institution, and ever be financially solvent again, there were specific amends to be made. I had to be honest and cooperative, work my recovery program, test clean, and empty my retirement accounts to pay financial amends. In retrospect, I can say that those were the simple direct amends on my list. Do this, answer and sign that, make those daily calls, go here and there, and in two to five years, this chapter of my life would be closed. This was all spelled out for me before I ever worked any of the steps. Those amends were about my transgressions against the rules of society, against the unseen entities that I hid from all those using years.

My remaining amends, as I came to understand through working Steps Four and Five, were about my personal relationships, those direct, person-to-person contacts of my entire past life. Whether I felt like a victim or a victimizer, it was important for me to take action to resolve the damage done. I would never feel like a whole spiritual person without taking those actions. Making amends helped me repair the relationship I have with God—that part of my spiritual nature that I hold sacred. Ridding myself of as much of that emotional baggage as possible would afford me some serenity—something I would need to lessen my chances of using pills again.

The easiest person to include on my amends list was, of course, me. But if I ever wanted to forgive myself, I would have to learn to forgive and understand my family members whose actions I believe drove me to my pill addiction. Through a family member's slip of the tongue, I found out that the father I always assumed was Dad was not my biological father. I was the big family secret, the result of an affair between my mother and the pastor of our church. I felt the full range of emotions—from betrayal and hatred to a sort of acceptance—and I thought, "Oh, that explains a lot."

All three of my parents took this secret to their graves. With the encouragement and support of my sponsor and a lot of prayer, I sought information from my remaining family members. Most refused to discuss the matter with me, but I finally found a relative who was forthcoming. Although difficult to hear, I was grateful for his honesty. It helped me accept the past and feel like I had some closure on the situation. I came to understand how the family dynamic of a broken marriage that was never dissolved affected me. I cannot recall seeing my parents drink or use drugs. Instead, I believe they used me. I was their drug, the cement that held together the dysfunction. I learned to survive on my own. I learned to play the system in my family. I became a double agent in my own home.

As I worked through this issue with my sponsor, I began to understand that my family didn't consciously or intentionally do this to me. It was just the way it was. They did the best they could, just as I had up until that point. It's taken some time and several graveside conversations, but it was important and beneficial for me to practice forgiveness in this particular situation.

I will say this about the Eighth Step experience and process: Admitting my wrongs to God, to another person, and to myself was the easy part. Talking directly with the injured parties was a little more involved.

Needless to say, I had formed some dysfunctional attitudes about relationships. The remainder of my amends list was occupied by the people I loved the most, my family. They were the ones most affected by my acting out. I owed a debt of gratitude to them, and not only spoken or written amends, but also the daily amends of going the extra mile to be the kind of husband, father, and person I always wanted to be.

As I remember, when I started taking pills, my world began to shrink. The more pills I used, the smaller my world became. Pills became my primary relationship, my friend, my lover, my God. I felt like it was unconditional love. Now

I realize that it was very conditional. For every pill I took I wrote a check against my future, my relationships, my body, and my spirit—and it felt like they all came due at once. I moved farther and farther away from my Higher Power, my family, friends, and co-workers. When I had conversations, I focused my eyes on that person, but mentally I was looking through them to the next high, or looking behind myself, running from the fear.

The amends I needed to make were not only for wrong actions or decisions, but also for the absence of actions or decisions. Emotional absenteeism or apathy caused my relationships to stagnate or die altogether. A lot of times I thought that the people I loved were unimportant, or simply in the way. When I got clean, I found myself feeling a lot of guilt and shame about this. I woke up in a world where my loved ones feared me and didn't trust me. In their place, I knew I would have felt the same. Even though I was under the influence, I could remember their reactions to some of the things I said and did.

My Eighth Step list has been valuable to me over the years. Whenever those old feelings of fear and resentment surface, I refer back to this list. Doing that helps me refocus my thinking from the problem to the solution. I have to accept the past as it was, wrong and unchangeable. With the help of P.A., I don't have to accept today or the future on that basis.

I LISTENED TO MY HEART AND NOT MY HEAD

Make a list of all persons I had harmed? Easy. I grabbed my Fourth Step list and showed up at my sponsor's house to do Step Nine. When she asked me why I brought my Fourth Step list, I was confused because someone told me that the Fourth Step list is the Eighth Step list. My sponsor had a different theory and practice. She asked me what "harming" another person meant, and I realized I had no idea, so I had to write out a definition. I stumbled and wrote something down that was way off base. She told me to read about the Eighth Step and show up the next week. I agreed, but I left feeling rather deflated and embarrassed.

Once I read about the step, I immediately saw my mistake. The Fourth Step is a good beginning for the list of all persons I had harmed, but many people were not listed; in fact, the only people listed were ones I resented. After doing my Fifth Step, I could clearly see how I had wronged those people. But for the Eighth Step, I had to think about all the people I had harmed throughout my life. I got clean at a later age, so I had a lot of life to think about. Listing those I had recently harmed was easy, but going back through my life was rather painful. I had to honestly ask myself who I had harmed physically, emotionally, mentally, financially, spiritually, or in any other way. As I thought back, my defenses charged in to protect me. I thought about an employee I had locked out of his office because I was too chicken to fire him. My mind immediately chimed in that he was a lousy employee, so I was right to lock him out. Self-justification became my working mode as I thought about my past, so I listed only a few people. After all, I was harmed more than many others were!

My sponsor pointed out that I was being totally self-centered and twisting the past to justify my behavior. She advised me to list all those I had harmed, regardless of whether they had harmed me, too. Working Step Eight wasn't about comparing how much I had wronged them to how much they had wronged me. I was *only* to think about how I had harmed others and put their names on the list.

But while I was making this list, I remembered the Ninth Step. There was no way I was going to list my brother. He had hurt me deeply as a teenager and had done terrible things to our family. Besides, I reasoned, I had never harmed him. So I left him off the list, reasoning that I didn't need his name for my Ninth Step list. After all, I figured that the purpose of

97

the Eighth Step list was really the list of people to whom we would do amends in the Ninth Step.

Again, my sponsor sent me back to put *everyone* on my list without filtering, justifying, or analyzing. She told me to stop being so analytical about it, and just list anyone I had harmed. Finally, I got it. I listened to my heart, not my head, and listed everyone I had harmed. Then I was hit with what felt like a Mack Truck of guilt and remorse. I couldn't believe how many people I had hurt. I thought that the only people I hurt were the ones who had to deal with me when I was high. But my list dated back to when I was nine years old and had been cruel to another child who shared a cabin with me at camp. I remembered not showing up at a wedding in which I was the maid of honor. I thought about employers I harmed by showing up high at work and not being as productive as I could have been, or worse yet, just calling in sick because I was having withdrawal pains or was too high to show up. The list went on and on.

When I sat down to read my list to my sponsor, I told her that I felt terrible about hurting these people. She told me that I should, but that, yet again, I was thinking about myself when I should be thinking about how to right my wrongs. At the end of reading my Eighth Step list, she asked me who I had left off the list. When I told her about my brother, she told me to pray for God to reveal to me how I had hurt my brother. It came instantly: I had not called to tell him about our mother's death. He found out from people who had read the obituaries and were calling him to offer their condolences. How could I have forgotten that? I wrote his name on my Eighth Step list. I saw how my disease had manifested at an early age, even before I ever took a pill, and how I had harmed many, many people. I was ready to do my Ninth Step.

Working this step took my honesty to a deeper level. After many years of being clean, I still remember situations, long buried in the past, in which I hurt another person. Now, I have my Ninth and Tenth Steps to right those wrongs. I am grateful that this Program has given me a design for living that works in all situations.

WORKING STEP EIGHT

With the Eighth Step, we complete the thorough self-examination we began in Step Four. In this crucial step, we list the individuals we have knowingly or unknowingly harmed, and describe the exact nature of the damage we caused. We review our list with our sponsor, and then pray for the willingness to make our amends to those we harmed, including ourselves. Answering the following questions, with the guidance of our sponsor, can help us to understand the wrongs we have done and muster the necessary courage to make the appropriate amends.

1. Why have I been reluctant to begin this step? What are some of my fears?

2. What other things get in the way of making amends (for example: shame, pride, justification, resentments)? What else?

3. Why is determining the exact nature of my wrongs important in the Eighth Step?

4. What are the different types of harm that I have caused? Have I included everything from the obvious harms, such as stealing, dishonesty, and physical abuse, to the more subtle types, such as abandonment and neglect?

5. As I list the resentments that stand in the way of my willingness to make amends, can I let these resentments go for now? If not, can I scrape together the willingness to add these names to my list anyway and work toward becoming willing later? With the help of

my sponsor, can I prioritize them according to their importance?

6. What are some of the things I have done to become willing? How do I feel about praying for willingness?

7. Why is it important to include myself on my list?

8. Why should I consult with my sponsor if there is anyone I am not sure about including on my list?

9. Why is it important not to rush things and try to make amends before consulting with my sponsor? What are the possible consequences?

10. Am I beginning to feel more connected with others and the world around me as the result of working this step? Am I beginning to feel compassion and empathy for others and myself? Describe.

STEP NINE

"Made direct amends to such people wherever possible, except when to do so would injure them or others."

Spiritual Principles: Forgiveness, Courage, Humility

We continue actively working our program of recovery in Step Nine. We have been preparing ourselves for this step since we began our journey. We have been learning about and practicing the principles of honesty, courage, and humility. We will draw from these character traits as we begin the next task before us. We recall from Step Eight that to amend is to improve, correct, remedy, or repair. By making amends, we are doing what is ours to do—cleaning up our side of the street and mending the wreckage caused by our behavior.

Fears and unrealistic expectations about Step Nine may be natural for us; however, mentally projecting about the making or outcome of our amends is time wasted and is detrimental to our purpose. We have learned in our work on Steps Six and Seven how our negative character traits have proven to be our downfall. This is no truer than when we contemplate making our amends. We will do well to remain focused and to avoid getting too caught up in fear: false evidence appearing real. Returning to Steps Two and Three will help us stay in the proper frame of mind. We are availed of a power greater than ourselves who will direct and guide us.

We must remember that we can only take responsibility for our own previous actions and for our own attempts to repair the damage we caused. We are not in control of outcomes or another person's reaction to our amends. What we offer to those we have harmed may be received in any number of ways. We do not need to be forgiven or pardoned by those to whom we make amends. Knowing this, we can be prepared mentally and spiritually. Ultimately, we make our amends and leave the results in the hands of our Higher Power.

Before addressing each person or institution on our Eighth Step list, we check our motives and intentions. Are we harboring traces of self-centeredness by hoping for a return amends from the person we are approaching? Are we searching for clemency without any real remorse? Are we only making our amends to rekindle an old relationship? Having worked through the steps to this point has given us clearer vision. We can now see the misdeeds of our past with greater clarity and identify situations in which we have caused harm that we may have previously overlooked. With our renewed sense of dignity and humility, we develop a genuine desire to set things right. We also have a profound desire to be free of guilt (I *did* something bad) and shame (I *am* something bad). Through the Twelve Steps, we have been given the tools to make these desires a reality.

Our sponsor's help and guidance will once again be invaluable. Before each amends, we discuss the process with him or her. We want to avoid clearing our conscience at the risk of creating more harm, either to another or to ourselves. Our sponsor will help us look at the person we harmed, the reason for the amends, and how we are actually going to make the amends. We have learned that, left to our own best thinking, we often found ourselves in trouble. We are now in the embrace of a new way of living that involves sharing our thoughts and ideas with someone we trust.

Many of our amends will be made directly, but there may be circumstances that prevent this. Death or distance may not allow us to meet those we have harmed face-to-face. A letter written to one who has died may be a powerful way to heal. For those who are unattainable because of distance, a phone conversation may serve the purpose. Situations such as these are discussed with our sponsor. It is important to remember that a person is not taken off the list because they are not physically available.

There may be those on our list to whom we have committed grave wrongs, such as permanent physical or emotional damage, or even death. We may face legal and financial consequences as a result of our past behaviors. We look at these circumstances individually with the help of our sponsor and our Higher Power. We ask and pray for guidance in how to proceed, knowing that we are not alone. We will be provided all that we need as long as we are honest and willing.

Making amends to those who have also harmed us can sometimes be difficult. In these situations we may still harbor so much resentment that we cannot bring ourselves to make the necessary amends. However, our program teaches us that when we have been harmed, we must practice the spiritual principle of forgiveness. Although it may seem impossible to even imagine at first, some of us have found that praying for the person we resent has softened our hearts and changed our perspective. Asking for others to enjoy the health, happiness, and prosperity we want for ourselves frees us from the bitterness of resentment and allows compassion and understanding to direct our thoughts and actions. Through prayer and thorough application of the previous steps, we can find it in our hearts to forgive those who harmed us, and become willing to make our amends to them in the same way we would to anyone else.

When faced with completing particularly challenging amends, we may find ourselves slipping into procrastination or avoidance. In Step Seven, we humbly asked the God of our understanding to remove these shortcomings. We can again call on what we have learned in this and previous steps for the strength to move forward. We pray for willingness and courage. When we are ready to make our amends, we keep our message simple and personal. We need not grovel or belittle ourselves before the people or institutions we have harmed. We have done much work to uncover and rediscover our true nature. We carry ourselves with a spirit of humility, knowing we are not the best of the best or the worst of the worst. We have done the footwork and we are ready.

Step Nine is not just about making amends, it is about living our amends. In the past, we said we were sorry many times, only to repeat the same behavior again and again. Today, we are living life free from the clutches of active addiction and self-obsession. We strive to adopt an attitude of service and steer clear of past harmful behaviors. One of the most powerful offerings we can make in reparation to others and society is to continue our journey of recovery, using the spiritual tools of our program to guide our way. Similarly, one of the best ways we can make amends to ourselves is through the living amends of our new, fulfilling lifestyle.

Our step work will leave us with a true sense of freedom. Our perspective on life will soften. We have faced our past honestly, thoroughly, and courageously. Regret for the past falls away as we now see that no matter what we have done or where we have been, we can use our experience to help others. All the trials, struggles, and defeats were not in vain because we can now share our experience with another suffering addict. Our world is becoming bigger as we exchange self-seeking behaviors for acts of service. Our feelings of worthlessness disappear as we find purpose in helping others. We begin to see fear as forgetting everything's all right, and we realize that fear no longer has the power to paralyze us. We know serenity for we have experienced it deep within. Grace and inspiration replace turmoil as we move through circumstances that used to trap us. A seemingly unexplainable and comforting sense of direction and certainty is guiding our lives today. We have stepped aside and allowed a power greater than ourselves to orchestrate our lives and lead us through each day. We feel the eternal flow of goodness in and around us. Life is full of promise. We are free to move forward with renewed confidence, self-respect, and joy.

OUR MEMBERS' EXPERIENCE WITH STEP NINE

THE REWARDS ARE BETTER THAN THE TORMENT OF REGRET

My journey into pill addiction started in my teens when I gave myself permission to take just about any mind-altering substance in pill or other form to escape from the reality of painful emotions. After an almost-fatal accident and spiritual experience in my mid-twenties, I managed to stay relatively abstinent for several years without any kind of recovery program.

During the next ten years, I developed physical problems as a result of the accident. These physical problems magnified my inability to cope with the pressures of raising two young children, dealing with an unemployed spouse, and having to return to work. I started to sneak wine under the pretense that I was using it for cooking. After a period of controlled drinking and using over-the-counter medications, I changed doctors. Lo and behold, I got what I was looking for —a drug that would help me sleep and make it easier for me to cope with life.

My pain and anxiety got worse, of course, and I had many symptoms that were treated with pills and surgeries. I devised numerous ways to "need" more procedures and surgeries because I knew I would get more pills. Over a period of ten years I lost the ability to work, to drive a car, and to care for my family or myself. Because I had so many surgeries, I had everyone convinced that I needed help with everything. I manipulated and conned everyone, told lies about my husband to gain sympathy, and in the end, I had only a few friends left. My family wanted nothing to do with me except my fourteen-year-old daughter who helped care for me. After my last bout in the hospital, I ended up in a nursing home. My sixteen-year-old son cried at my bedside, saying how he remembered who I used to be and how vibrant and happy I had been. With the help of a counselor, I was given the choice to either go into recovery or have my medications administered to me. Although I didn't know about it at the time, my husband had arranged with a lawyer to have me committed if I refused.

I surrendered and went to treatment and halfway houses for the next eight months. It was very difficult as I had to face my physical and emotional pain without pills. During this time, I started working the steps with a sponsor, found a home group, and helped to start a P.A. meeting. Through working the steps, I found out that fear and self-centeredness had ruled my life and that I harmed many people as a result. I made a list of the people I had harmed. It was a long list and I was afraid, but I had gained strength from working the previous steps, which included a renewed and much-improved relationship with a loving God. My sponsor suggested that I start with my family and the other people I had harmed the most.

I remember each amends to this day and where each one took place. With my sponsor's help, I kept my amends short and to-the-point, accepting full responsibility without excuses for the harm I had done, and asking what I could do to right my wrongs. Once I did my first several amends I felt a burden lifted and I was energized to go on. I remember making amends to my ninety-six-year-old grandmother for lying to her to get a large sum of money, which she deducted from my inheritance as retribution. As part of my amends to my husband, I asked him to be present when I made amends to many of my church friends. I did this because I had lied to them about him, and couldn't remember what I had said to which people because I was often in a blackout.

My life changed as a result of making amends, even though several people told me they could never trust me again. Living amends, especially with my family, helped me gradually regain their trust. I was becoming free from the guilt, shame, and remorse of my past. I still occasionally make amends as my memory returns because I know the rewards are so much better than the torment of regret.

Admitting My Part Changed My Life

My Ninth Step story goes something like this. In Step Eight I made a list of the people I had wronged. On that list was an ex-wife. We had separated some twenty-three years earlier, and then divorced three years later. I felt I owed her an amends because the divorce wasn't all her fault. I did have a part in it. I saw her email address on an email one of my daughters had sent me and I didn't know her phone number, so after talking it over with my sponsor, we decided an email would be okay. I sent an email saying basically that when we were married (and after), I had acted and behaved wrongly. I wrote that I had done things that would hurt anyone—and she was that person. I explained that I knew I could not change what I had done, but I wanted to make things right. I only talked about my part in it, not even trying to bring up her faults. The email message was all me and my behaviors.

When she wrote back, she said she was glad I saw that I had a part in the relationship ending, and that we were both young at the time and not to fret over the past.

But the other thing that happened was that she gave my daughters permission to openly talk about me and speak directly to me, instead of hiding our communications as they had done for years. My oldest daughter called me one day shortly after that saying she was going to be in a neighboring state for a week and wanted to meet me. I said I could fly over and meet her.

We had not seen each other in more than twenty-one years. When the day came, I was very nervous—outright afraid. What if she only wanted to tell me off to my face, tell me she hated me? A lot of people from my home group talked to me on the phone that day. They talked to me before I went to the airport, while I was waiting for the plane, and when I finally landed.

I got off the plane and made my way to the baggage area when I suddenly realized I didn't know what she looked like. How would I know her? I neared the escalators that went down to the baggage claim area, wondering what I was going to do. As I stepped onto the escalator, I looked down below and there she was—a young lady holding a cardboard sign that said, "DAD."

We hugged, we cried, we hugged some more. It was beautiful. I could never have believed this would have happened in a million years. We had lunch on a pier over the ocean and then went back to the airport. It was Friday evening and I was two hours late for my flight, but I didn't care. I was on top of the world.

I met my other daughter eleven months later when she attended my wedding. It was really nice to be together after such a long time. It would never have happened if I hadn't worked the steps and had a spiritual transformation. Before that, I was so sure others had done all of the harm to me, and that I was just a victim. In the end, when I saw and admitted my part, my life changed.

WORKING STEP NINE

Having accepted responsibility for the harm we caused, and having developed some willingness to right those wrongs, we now tackle the gut-wrenching, yet deeply rewarding Ninth Step. To everyone listed in Step Eight, we make direct amends wherever possible and, when necessary, we make indirect amends. We are always careful not to cause any further harm in the process. We have found that honestly and thoroughly answering the following questions and frequently consulting with our sponsor are of inestimable value in the completion of Step Nine.

1. What is the purpose of Step Nine and how will it benefit my recovery and peace of mind?

2. How is making amends more than just verbally making an apology (like saying, "I am sorry.")?

3. Have I thoroughly discussed with my sponsor, and possibly another person in recovery, my list of amends and how to proceed with the amends process?

4. How can my Higher Power, my sponsor, and other recovering pill addicts be a source of strength in this process?

5. Am I spiritually prepared for making any difficult amends, and for dealing with the consequences? What have I done to prepare myself?

6. What types of changes or restitution (i.e. financial, behavioral, or living) am I willing and able to put into action to correct my wrongs?

7. What expectations do I have of how other people will receive my amends, and am I willing to turn those expectations over to my Higher Power?

8. How can I make up for the wreckage and pain I caused in the past, to my loved ones and myself, through living amends?

9. To whom do I make direct amends?

10. How will I make amends to those I have tried unsuccessfully to find?

11. What kinds of amends can be made when a person has died?

12. What types of amends are those I cannot make without harming others? How can I make these amends anonymously to avoid hurting innocent people?

13. Are there any amends I want to make anonymously rather than directly? Have I discussed these with my sponsor?

14. Which amends am I procrastinating about and why? Are fears of personal embarrassment, financial loss, or loss of freedom holding me back? How has this stood in the way of my recovery?

STEP TEN

"Continued to take personal inventory and when we were wrong promptly admitted it."

Spiritual Principles: Discipline, Vigilance, Honesty

Step Ten is about developing a continued awareness of our behaviors, thoughts, and emotions. We have worked diligently to clear the wreckage of our past. We have acquired a sense of freedom that lifts us up and feeds our desire for this new way of living. We can no longer afford to be unaware of our behavior and attitudes, and how they affect us and those around us. We will want to keep our house in order so we can maintain this newfound serenity along with our continued recovery.

In Steps Four through Nine we reviewed our past, discussed it with another person, asked our Higher Power to remove our character defects, and made amends to those we had harmed. In working Step Ten, we employ the same practices on a daily basis. We want to prevent the debris of resentments, self-pity, and self-deception from accumulating so it does not harm us or others. This requires honest self-searching and reflection. Our motives may not always be apparent at first glance. We may have to look deeply to discover if we have been driven by fear, selfishness, dishonesty, or self-righteousness. It takes discipline to be open-minded and admit we have not been justified in our thinking or actions. However, the payoff far exceeds the effort, for we have long experienced the symptoms of emotional hangovers: unease, restlessness, irritability, and depression. These are the symptoms we ran from, searching for a bottle of pills to ease our pain. We now know a better way of living, and Step Ten allows us to stay in balance by maintaining our emotional and mental health.

We cannot and must not become complacent with this step. Failure to take personal inventory on a regular, daily basis will eventually find us experiencing an undercurrent of discontent. The symptoms we turned to pills to escape from will creep back into our lives to haunt us. Irritability, depression, fear, and insidious anxiety will replace our sense of well-being. Finding fault and passing judgment begin to rob us of our serenity and peace of mind. Control, expectations, and resentment form a Bermuda Triangle that threatens to suck us under. Mental and emotional binges lead to spiritual blackouts, leaving us vulnerable and susceptible to relapse.

Like any exercise, with daily practice we will soon find our efforts paying off. With time and perseverance, the healthy habit of taking a daily inventory will become part of our lives. What once seemed impossible to remember or put to use will become second nature to us. We become watchful for the emergence of old thoughts and behavior patterns that can build into waves of destruction. Better to stop a trickle than fight a torrent. When we are tempted to react, we learn to hit the pause button. We step back and think it through. Our response will then have a greater chance of being in the best interests of all concerned. Our vigilance will be rewarded. We will find ourselves becoming more adept at listening to the voice of intuition, our gut feelings. We will be acutely aware whenever our inner balance is upset. The accompanying feeling of discomfort will be our cue to become still and take stock of our actions, intentions, perceptions, and self-seeking desires.

When emotions run high, intelligence tends to take a back seat. We run the risk of regret, self-condemnation, and strained or broken relationships when we indulge in emotional extremes. Having tasted freedom, we are no longer content with feeling trapped in such negative states of being. We are motivated to change what needs changing and preserve what is working. By working the steps we have acquired many tools for improving the quality of our lives. Drama and chaos no longer have such a strong appeal for us. Kindness, love, and acceptance have replaced self-centeredness. We are striving for harmony within and with others. We have demonstrated the courage to take care of ourselves. Step Ten is our continued commitment to our recovery journey.

Often, we find our sponsor's insight to be of great value to us when working this step. Our own vision can be short-sighted. We may not see the truth of a situation because of our misperceptions. We may not be able to honestly see our part in certain circumstances. With the help of another person, a different perspective may be revealed, one unclouded by emotional intensity. When we find we were wrong, we admit it, first to ourselves and to our Higher Power, and then to whomever else might be involved. We are familiar by now with humility. We need not fear making amends, because we now know this practice helps us maintain our emotional balance and leads to our continued peace of mind. We set things right as soon as possible. We use the discernment and consideration we employed when making our amends in Step Nine. When in doubt, we connect with the wisdom and guidance of our sponsor.

We will also find ourselves faced with wrongs done to us by others. These real or perceived wrongs may be a grave injustice, or a minor annoyance. To maintain our balance, we practice love, tolerance, patience, and forgiveness. We remember that we have been spiritually sick, and how in our disease we brought pain into other people's lives. In this spirit, we find compassion for others who may also be spiritually ailing. We remember that we are all at different stages of spiritual growth on our separate journeys.

We try to practice Step Ten as we go through our day and then do a more thorough inventory at day's end. We may conduct our review mentally or in writing, but in either case we consider whether we have consistently worked the principles of our program throughout the day. Were we responsible with our obligations? Did we treat those we encountered with kindness and respect? Have we been of service? Did we stay clean today? Our inventory should take into account all aspects of our day. Actively practicing Step Ten throughout the course of our day, we watch for self-centeredness, dishonesty, resentment, and fear, pausing to ask God to remove them. We discuss any mental, emotional, or spiritual *dis*-ease with someone we trust, and make necessary amends as soon as possible. Being of service will help to keep us from getting stuck in destructive thoughts. We want to avoid mentally thrashing ourselves for errors. We are not spiritually perfect. Step Ten is an opportunity to examine "what is" and make corrections where necessary.

Tomorrow is a brand new day and a chance to once again put into practice the tools, behaviors, and attitudes we have learned from working the program of Pills Anonymous. We are thankful for the many blessings we have received in our recovery from pill addiction. We see that the more we adopt an attitude of gratitude, the easier it is to stay on the beam of recovery. This is spiritual growth. In this we persevere, one day at a time.

Our Members' Experience with Step Ten

A Victim No More

At first glance, Step Ten intimidated me because it suggested that I turn the lens inward and look honestly at myself. It recommended that at all times, regardless of anyone else's role or actions, I should take responsibility for my life. It suggested I was not a victim and that I was in charge of maintaining my happiness, and that when I was disturbed, it was because something was wrong *with me.*

All of my life I thought I was a victim of my surroundings. I was justified in my anger because *he* didn't take my feelings into account, or I wasn't at fault because *she* started it, or you would be nicer to me if only you knew me better... I lived my life feeling that I was at the whim of everyone else's selfish desires. When someone hurt me, I would do what I had to do to protect myself, whether that was to yell back, withhold love, or secretly plot my revenge. I spent a great deal of time angry, sad, and lonely because I really thought no one liked me. Those feelings were always worse at night when it was just me, alone with my thoughts. Many nights I would try to fall asleep, but I couldn't because I had a turning knot in the pit of my stomach and a deep ache in my chest.

Even after I got clean, I experienced these feelings for a while. After my Fifth Step I began the process of forgiving and accepting myself, and the sleepless nights started getting better. It wasn't until after my Ninth Step that the ache was really lifted from my chest completely. I realized that the negative feelings didn't come from other people not liking me as I had always suspected. They actually came from *me* not liking me.

I spent a while with a new peace and serenity I had never known, but in time the old familiar ache was back. I had been free of it, but it was back! Where were my Ninth Step promises of freedom, confidence, self-respect, and joy? I knew something had to change, and I thought I was willing to do what was needed to ensure my emotional serenity.

I expressed my concerns to my sponsor and immediately felt better when she nodded and smiled. I recounted a tale of my unfair boss making unreasonable demands on me that led me to feel terrible afterwards. As with many other confrontational situations I had been involved in, I was pretty sure it was the other person's fault, that if I explained my feelings to them and asked them to treat me differently, I would feel better. Imagine my surprise when my sponsor asked me what *my* part was in all of it!

This was my introduction to the Tenth Step. My sponsor told me that my next stage of recovery was for me to grow in understanding and effectiveness through a continual process of improving upon who I am, how I act, and how I can be of service. She explained that a great way to do that would be to become aware of how I respond to situations that anger me. I began at that time to take the Tenth Step into my daily life. When I was upset, I learned to respond first by asking myself where I was at fault. Normally I ask myself, "Where was I selfish, dishonest, resentful, or afraid?" When I identify one of those, I ask God to remove it right away. Then I talk it over with someone to see where and if I owe amends, I make those amends, and then I directly get into being of service to someone else. This last step is crucial for me to avoid both morbid self-reflection *and* further self-centeredness.

I understand today that in order to keep growing toward God (and away from using), I have to keep taking this daily personal inventory. In order to maintain my spiritual serenity today, I always have to look at my own behavior, and focus on keeping my side of the street clean. When I slack on this step and begin thinking I need to take other people's inventories instead of my own, I start to lose my connection with God. As a guideline, I take a quick inventory anytime I am upset or feel like I may have upset someone else, as well as at the end of the day. When I started using this tool I really started maturing as a person.

Every day that I wake up not needing to take a pill is a gift from God, and that gift is dependent upon me working to be the most loving and helpful person I can be. Today I live a very blessed life and I genuinely love my fellow human beings and myself. I think the gift of this step is that I am able to decide my own level of happiness. I am a victim no more.

A LINT ROLLER FOR RESENTMENTS

After ten years clean (preceded by two relapses over a seven-year period), I was becoming complacent. I attended at least five meetings a week, called my sponsor daily, had multiple sponsees myself, and thought I was working a good program. I have long had chronic pain as a result of car accidents and sports injuries, and it was that pain which first led me to pills. But in my long-term clean time, I learned to manage that pain fairly well, and take care of myself when it flared up. Yet, one day, when I was in pain, it suddenly made perfect sense to me to help myself to some of my (non-addict) wife's pain medication—and then to do so again several times over the weeks to come, before (thank God) I felt so nauseous with guilt and remorse that I cancelled a business trip and declared my relapse to my wife, to my sponsor, and to my fellow pill addicts in recovery.

I couldn't understand what had gone wrong. Why had I made that foolish choice? I had previously endured worse pain without using mind-altering medications. I also knew that if such medication was truly necessary, the recovery-based approach would be to speak to my doctor, my sponsor, and other fellow P.A. members before making such a decision.

At the request of my shocked and angry wife, I spent two weeks "living elsewhere" while she dealt with her feelings about my deception and theft, with the help of her twelve-step program for the families and friends of addicts. During the second week of this separation, while attending a meeting, I suddenly heard a loud voice in my head saying "You haven't been working the Tenth Step!"

I sat there stunned. The Tenth Step had not been a topic of discussion in that meeting, and yet at that moment it was absolutely clear to me that I had just received a message from my Higher Power. My jaw dropped, because what I had heard throughout my recovery was quite accurate. Despite continuously attending twelve-step meetings for many years, and despite working the steps, the fact was that I did not practice the Tenth Step as it was outlined in our guiding literature. I didn't write about my resentments, my fears, etc., on a daily basis, and I am a lint roller for resentments. Little resentments that probably stretched back to the beginning of my clean time had been allowed to build and build until even a small resentment immediately evolved into a big one. It was then that I admitted to myself that it wasn't physical pain which motivated me to take the meds. It was the emotional pain associated with the resentments I had against the person I loved and cherished most, my wife.

Since that day, a written daily Tenth Step has become the linchpin of my program. I write it in an email which I send to my sponsor, and I save a copy in an email folder I call "GB." That's right; I'm a geek with an electronic "God Box." It works for me. The sense of freedom I have as a result of working *all* the steps is amazing. And, once again, I realized that if I give my disease of addiction *any* opening, it will try to kill me. I am grateful that I (and my marriage) survived.

WORKING STEP TEN

With Step Ten, we commit ourselves to the lifelong process of maintaining our recovery by applying Steps Four through Nine to our lives on a regular basis. For Step Ten, many of us find it useful to make a list of our personal strengths and weaknesses. At the beginning or end of each day we review this list and honestly appraise our actions over the last twenty-four hours. We note the occasions when we were successful in applying the spiritual principles of recovery in our daily lives, and we also admit when we have fallen short of our spiritual goals. We promptly admit our mistakes. Whenever our shortcomings have caused harm, we make amends, relying on the guidance of our sponsor and our own experience in working Step Nine.

1. Why is it important for me to continue taking action each and every day to maintain my self-awareness and spiritual condition?

2. How has promptly admitting my wrongs helped me become aware of, and continue to change, my behavior?

3. Why is it important to continue taking a personal inventory on a daily basis and what might I achieve through this practice? What can I do to make sure that after a period of time a daily inventory will become second nature?

4. When and how do I seek guidance from my Higher Power in working Step Ten? How often do I seek guidance from my sponsor?

5. What are the items I have included on my checklist of positive and negative character traits?

The following questions may be used as a daily Tenth Step checklist

1. How was I kind and loving to the people I encountered today?

2. In what ways was I selfish, dishonest, or afraid?

3. If I set myself up for disappointment, what contributed to this? Was it because of unrealistic expectations?

4. Did I allow myself to become hungry, angry, lonely, or tired by not managing my life well? If so, in what ways?

5. If I am taking things—or myself—too seriously in any area of my life, how did this show up in my perceptions, thoughts, or behavior?

6. Did I feel any fear in my life today? What about?

7. Did I experience any extreme feelings today? Which ones? To what was I responding and why did I have these feelings?

8. Did I feel disturbed about something and not share it with my sponsor or another recovering pill addict? How can secrets build up and cause difficulty with my clean time?

9. Was there anything I did today that I felt I should not have done? Were there things I did not do today that I felt I should have done? What were these things?

10. Did I stay true to my personal integrity in all my relationships today?

11. Did I experience conflicts in any of my relationships today? What were they and who did they involve? How could I have behaved differently?

12. On occasions when I did not do the right thing, what could I have done differently? How can I do it better at the next opportunity?

13. Do I owe amends to anyone because of my behavior today? When and how can I make those amends?

14 What are some of the things I have done today that I feel positive about, and that have given me satisfaction? Do I want to be sure I repeat these actions?

15. How does practicing self-discipline in this step affect my recovery and my life?

16. Did I take care of myself by going to a meeting or talking to another recovering pill addict today? Was I of service to another person today?

17. What are some of the things I am especially grateful for today?

STEP ELEVEN

"Sought through prayer and meditation to improve our conscious contact with God, as we understood Him, praying only for knowledge of His will for us and the power to carry that out."

Spiritual Principles:
Persistence, Open-Mindedness, Discipline, Humility

As we continue to live a life of recovery, we adopt another daily practice. We are learning to let go of our self-destructive behaviors and time-consuming obsessions. We make a conscious effort now to fill that space with a relationship with a Higher Power. We began building this relationship in Step Two when we acknowledged a power greater than our own. In Step Three, although it took a leap of faith for some of us, we began to trust the God of our understanding. In Step Eleven, we continue along this spiritual pathway, developing a channel of communication with this power that guides us.

We have achieved abstinence from pills by staying clean one day at a time. In looking back, we can easily see our progress in maintaining recovery. If we pause to consider our spiritual progress, we will see that we have also grown in this regard. In the same way that we stay clean one day at a time, we have a daily reprieve from mental and emotional whirlpools if we maintain our spiritual condition. As our physical, mental, and emotional well-being improves, so do our lives. We find that we can handle, grow through, and even enjoy previously unmanageable and upsetting aspects of our lives.

However, without consistent attention to our spiritual life and communication with our Higher Power, we run the risk of thinking, "I have this thing licked, and can take it from here on my own." For this reason, we must remain alert for signs of complacency. Forgetting the powerlessness we discovered in Step One, allowing resentment and intolerance to take up residence, procrastinating on making amends, losing interest in fellow pill addicts (especially the newcomer), and allowing excuses to replace meeting attendance are all signs of straying from the path of recovery. When we return to self-will we are at serious risk of relapse. Step Eleven continues our maintenance program and is vital to our continued recovery.

We appeal to our open-mindedness when working Step Eleven. With a fair amount of investigation and experimentation, even the most skeptical of us have found results when practicing prayer and meditation. Many of us have come to understand that prayer is simply talking to God, and meditation is listening for God's answer. For those of us just beginning this practice, we have found that keeping it simple is good advice. Starting our recovery journey did not feel natural at first, yet we came to realize that with perseverance we became comfortable with our newfound principles and routines.

With the continued practice of Step Eleven, we will find the same to be true of prayer and meditation. No rules or dictates are set forth on exactly how we should proceed, but we may find and benefit from the guidance of our fellow members in Pills Anonymous. Listening to what others do and considering the many ways that others practice prayer and meditation will help us discover our own personal path. There is no right or wrong way to pray or meditate. Just as we have the right to form our own beliefs about our Higher Power, we have the same right to personalize our prayer and meditation. Our method and style remain as individual choices. We may try several variations before we settle on one that feels comfortable and right for us. The important thing is to persevere in our spiritual practice. Developing and expanding our relationship with our Higher Power provides us with mental and emotional nourishment and support.

We are cautious when asking for specifics in prayer. Why? When we decide what "should be" by requesting a specific outcome, we run the risk of being ego-centered and setting ourselves up for disappointment, creating expectations that may not be fulfilled. When we take back our will, we do not leave room for our Higher Power to move in our lives. We search our motivations and intentions, and if we do pray for a specific outcome, we humbly make our request, adding, "or as You see best." Although we have dreams and desires, we remain open to the possibility that God may want us to travel a different road.

When we are caught up in fear, doubt, conflict, or indecision, we can pause and spiritually reconnect by using a simple phrase or request. Taking a brief or extended timeout allows us to clear mental and emotional debris, opening a channel for grace and wisdom. We ask throughout our day for an understanding of our Higher Power's will for us and the power to carry it out. Consider this simple prayer:

> *Deliver me from ego, that I may be Your light in the world today. Be my words, guide my thoughts. Lead me to be love and laughter, joy and light, hope and harmony, peace and forgiveness, compassion and understanding, truth and wisdom.*

We may have big questions and concerns regarding God's will. How do we know our Higher Power's will? We have been practicing many spiritual principles since beginning our journey with the Twelve Steps. These principles emphasize integrity and respect for ourselves and others in our world. They emerge from an open heart and an attitude of kindness, acceptance, and gratitude. We create a certain level of energy when operating our lives according to these principles, an energy that produces inner peace and wisdom. It has been said that God's will for us is to replace shame, guilt, and fear with an inner serenity born of a life lived with love, dignity, joy, and service. As we become more familiar with our inner climate, we can use this as a compass to guide us in communicating with our Higher Power.

Starting and ending the day with an "attitude of gratitude" is a simple way to connect with our Higher Power. Many of us ask for the help to stay clean each morning and thank our Higher Power for the grace to do so when we lie down at night. Whatever amount of time we devote to Step Eleven, we strive for daily practice. In time, we will see this period we set aside for connecting with our Higher Power as an indispensable part of our lives, as essential to us as eating and breathing. It is a basic necessity for spiritual well-being. Most of us will notice an uncomfortable change in our emotional balance and mental peace of mind if we skip this vital part of our day.

Like our recovery, Step Eleven is a journey. As we begin to experience a deeper connection with our Higher Power, we try to remain open-minded. We may find our concept of our Higher Power changing as we grow in understanding. Just as our views of a friend have changed over the years since we first met, the same will be true as our relationship with our Higher Power grows. We need not fear surrendering to this unfolding. Just as a raindrop becomes a part of the ocean, we are surrounded and supported by an endless supply of courage, love, tolerance, and patience. We find that we are given whatever we need. We use our deepening relationship to serve as a channel of goodwill toward others.

By practicing this step, our old belief that we are victims of circumstance will be replaced with a new belief that we are empowered through our Higher Power. We will come to know that we are perfectly cared for at all times, in all things. All is well. With a renewed spirit we move on to Step Twelve.

OUR MEMBERS' EXPERIENCE WITH STEP ELEVEN

I GET EXACTLY WHAT I NEED

I've always considered myself a spiritual person. I grew up in a strict Catholic family, went to Sunday school every week, completed my Sacraments, and as I got older, I even taught Sunday school. There was never even a time in my life when I did not believe in a Higher Power. When I was abusing pills, I still prayed every day. I prayed that I would never wake up and that He would take me from this hell I considered life. I was angry with my Higher Power every time I woke up. "Why doesn't He take me and spare someone that has a life worth living?" I would ask.

After I first got clean, I continued to pray and meditate, but for different things. In my first ninety days I prayed that everyone would leave me alone, that my chronic pain would go away, and that I wouldn't have to go to these meetings anymore because I would be cured. During the rest of my first year clean, I prayed for a job, money, a cell phone, a boyfriend, and maybe a few new friends. And then in my second year clean, I prayed for peace in my heart, to be relieved of guilt and shame, and for love from my family and friends. Eventually, as I learned to live in recovery and work the Twelve Steps of Pills Anonymous, I prayed for the knowledge of God's will and the power to carry that out.

Today I realize it doesn't matter what I pray for because I will get exactly what I need and what He wants me to have. If I were to write out my wants (prayers) when I first got clean and all of them happened, I would be truly disappointed now. In recovery I have received many things I didn't know I needed and several things I didn't want at the time, but ended up grateful for in the end. When I was newly clean, I wasn't even capable of imagining all the wonderful things I would be given in recovery.

A good example of this is the relationship I had with my mother. For my entire life, she and I had never been particularly close. When I was in my twenties, my mom divorced my dad. I was so angry with her that I didn't want to speak to her for the rest of my life. I didn't speak to her for more than two years, even on her birthday and Christmas. I never wanted her in my life in any capacity. It wasn't until I had been clean for a couple of years that I started to come around. Working the Twelve Steps and seeking outside assistance helped me to realize that she was also an addict. She was sick like me. I started spending a little time with her. At first it was just lunch, after which I would immediately leave. A few months later we started going to garage sales and out for breakfast on Saturday mornings. I decided I wasn't going to try to make this relationship anything that I had in my mind. I prayed for God's will and the power to carry it out. Slowly, we reintegrated back into each other's lives. I was able to see through prayer and meditation that she was just a human being who loved, lost, felt pain, was hurt as a child, had unfulfilled dreams, and was only trying to live life the best way she knew how. I prayed every night for God to show me how to be the best possible daughter and friend to her. As time went on, and we worked on our relationship, I came to forgive my mom for the pain I felt. As a result, my pain lessened more and more. Today, I am overjoyed and proud to say I have a good relationship with my mom and I love her very much.

I FORGOT WHO I WAS

My pre-recovery version of Step Eleven could have been, "I sought through prayer and medication to improve my conscious contact with God..."

Yep, that's right. I tried medicine, religion, and psychiatry (separately and together), but none of these were sufficient to bring about a change in me that could only happen through conscious contact with the God of my understanding. Lack of a Higher Power had always been my dilemma in life.

My recovery journey began when I entered a treatment facility where I was introduced to the Twelve Steps. My goal was to stop using drugs and live life like "normal" people live it. I succeeded. I became a successful substance abuse counselor and program director over the next few years and showed everyone what a great person I had become. I could teach you how to change your life, help you solve your problems and guide you where you ought to go. What a great guy I was!

But there was a major problem lurking in the shadows: I quit working MY program. After several years of being clean, the once strong relationship I had with my Higher Power began to wane. I quit believing that God was in charge and slowly started to take back control of my life. That began the process of relapse for me. My meeting attendance was the next thing to suffer, and then I stopped contacting my sponsor and working the steps. I thought I was cured! I thought I could do it on my own. I was very wrong. The next three years would be the most devastating of my life.

I suffered from physical problems during that time, but I didn't address the problem until it became so bad that surgery was my only option. Post-surgery pain medication was prescribed for me and I will never forget the "head change" I received after popping that first pill. It truly woke up the "sleeping giant." The medication took me to a place to which

I thought I would never return. I took the medication as prescribed and when the pain was gone, so were the pills. I thought, "That wasn't so difficult." But that was only a form of self-deception, one that I didn't know was beginning to consume me. Just seven months later I found myself asking a friend for a few of his pills and that is what began my relapse after several years clean. I returned to full-blown addiction to prescription and street drugs. For the next year, I gave everything away to the disease—my family, home, career, and myself. I forgot who I was. I am an addict, and I know today that I will always be one.

After returning to the program, I realized that my recovery is dependent upon my conscious contact with a power greater than myself. That conscious contact comes through daily prayer and meditation (talking to God and listening for His answer). I go to Pills Anonymous meetings and fellowship with other pill addicts on a regular basis. I have a sponsor who I stay in contact with regularly. I am in service, and I work the steps. I know that these are the things I must do in order to stay clean.

WORKING STEP ELEVEN

Just as the Tenth Step prescribes a regular inventory to help sustain our recovery, Step Eleven suggests that prayer and meditation become an essential part of our daily routine. Many of us, inspired by the first three steps, our sponsors, and other recovering pill addicts, have begun to pray regularly and have experienced the benefits of improving our conscious contact with a God of our understanding. Step Eleven guides us in developing a more personal relationship with our Higher Power. Answering the following questions will help us form a deeper understanding of our Higher Power and how that power works in our lives. In working Step Eleven, as with all our steps, we rely on the experience, strength, and hope of our sponsor to guide us through any uncertainty and confusion we may have.

1. How have all the experiences I have had in recovery while working the steps, sharing with other recovering pill addicts, and practicing spiritual principles in my life, helped me to begin forming an understanding of what my Higher Power is like? What were those experiences? What did I come to believe in or understand about my Higher Power?

2. What characteristics and attributes do I believe my Higher Power has? How can I apply those qualities to my own life so that I can experience the changes my Higher Power has in store for me?

3. Have I come to believe there is a difference between spirituality and religion? What are those differences?

4. How does my relationship with Pills Anonymous help guide me on my spiritual journey?

5. What is my personal definition of prayer? How do I feel about praying? How and when do I pray?

6. How does praying steady my emotions and help me put life in perspective?

7. What is my definition of meditation? How do I feel about meditating? How and when do I meditate?

8. How do I feel when I am meditating, and do I see changes in myself as the result of these meditations?

9. In what situations have I been able to feel the presence of my Higher Power? How and what does it feel like?

10. What were the results when I made a conscious effort to align my will with God's will? What were some of the situations in which I surrendered my will?

11. What are some examples of what happened when I tried to run my life by my will alone?

12. Have I ever prayed for a specific thing, and after I received it, wished I did not have it after all? Have I ever prayed for something, not received it, and was later glad that I did not get what I so desperately wanted? Give examples.

13. How do I know the difference between my will and my Higher Power's will?

14. Why is humility essential for practicing Step Eleven?

15. What degree of commitment am I willing to make toward working Step Eleven on a regular basis, and how will I accomplish this?

STEP TWELVE

"Having had a spiritual awakening as the result of these steps, we tried to carry this message to addicts and to practice these principles in all our affairs."

Spiritual Principles:
Service, Generosity, Perseverance, Unconditional Love

Step Twelve brings it all together. It is the culmination of our work in each of the other Twelve Steps along the way. We have looked deeply at ourselves and we have done much to renew our inner spirit and self-respect. We have examined our relationships and taken the necessary steps to restore peace and harmony in our inner and outer worlds. We took risks knowing we had no control over outcomes, and that the only change we might effect would be within ourselves. As a result of our efforts, we slowly began to realize a gradual shift in our perceptions.

Many of us are not able to pinpoint the exact moment of our awakening. What we do experience is the dawning realization that we have undergone deep changes in the quality of our personalities. Before stepping into recovery, many of us were unaware of our Higher Power, did not know that we could access that power, and had no idea what that power could do in our lives. We could not possibly know the true miracles of recovery in the beginning, when all we could hope for was relief from the physical and mental agony of our active addiction. As we enter Step Twelve, we think back to all the times that a Higher Power has been at work within us, doing what we could not humanly do. No longer are we so easily irritated with the minor twists and turns of life. We are even able to handle major upheavals with grace and composure. We begin to see that we have choices in how we respond to people, places, and things. On a deep and personal level, we have learned and experienced forgiveness, acceptance, surrender, and trust. We are no longer confined to our own interests, ideas, needs, and wants. Today we see beyond self and respond to others. Compassion and tolerance are replacing impatience and resentment. We are given the courage and serenity to edge out fear and anxiety. Our past experience need not dictate or influence our present attitude and circumstances. It can, however, benefit others. Future and fear are no longer synonymous, as we now trust a power greater than ourselves to guide us and care for us.

Looking back, we are now aware of both who we were and who we have become. For some, this difference will be enormous, while for others it will be just a small beginning, but for all who continue this journey, much more will be revealed. The spiritual void in which we once lived is being filled, and we grow as a result.

Like tending a garden, we have found that to continue to reap the benefits, we must be vigilant in caring for our recovery. Working our program on a daily basis allows recovery to take root in our hearts and lives. When working with or serving others, we keep our recovery fresh by giving it away, and we reinforce our beliefs as we live the program. We get out of our own heads and discover the gift of helping another suffering pill addict. In assisting another person, we often find answers to the problems and dilemmas we face in our own lives. Sometimes, after reaching out to someone who is suffering, we find our own mental chaos and distress have disappeared altogether. More importantly, if we do not help others, we will use again. And if we use, we might die. Being of service and helping another pill addict is our greatest defense against taking that first pill.

There are many ways to serve others in the program. Volunteering for service positions helps maintain the stability of the Pills Anonymous group. Attending meetings, arriving early to greet people, and staying late to talk to fellow pill addicts can be done with any amount of recovery time. Helping to set up before the meeting and clean up afterwards are humble ways to serve the Pills Anonymous group. Attentive listening in meetings shows respect for fellow pill addicts, as does responsible sharing. Limiting how long we speak so others have enough time to share shows consideration and provides a welcoming atmosphere for the suffering pill addict. A friendly face and a warm welcome can be enough to make any pill addict walking through the doors for the first time feel safe. We remember what it was like for us, which inspires us to give away what we so freely received.

When sharing with another pill addict on a personal level, we have found it best to refrain from giving advice. We are not therapists, guidance counselors, financial advisors, personal affairs experts, or relationship gurus. What we have to give another is our experience, strength, and hope. We stick to this, for this is what we know best. We avoid the temptation to do for pill addicts what they can and should do for themselves. We carry the message, not the pill addict, allowing the newcomer to shoulder his or her own responsibilities. When a person comes to us with an honest desire for help, we share unconditionally, and without judgment. We have no special insight on who will grasp and hold onto this simple program of recovery. Our responsibility is to share what we have been given—what we have learned in life and in the program. We can ask the God of our understanding to be our guide. Carrying the message keeps us clean and also helps the suffering pill addict. Carrying the message is also important for the continuation of Pills Anonymous. We are responsible for the hand of Pills Anonymous to always be there, not only for the pill addict who suffers now, but for future pill addicts who will seek recovery.

What is the message that we carry? The spirit of our message is simply that, one day at a time, we do not have to take pills, and that we can lead lives that are happy, joyous, and free. We cannot do this alone. We have learned that life can be transformed when lived according to a few basic principles as found in the Twelve Steps of Pills Anonymous. We have learned to live in acceptance, openness, and humility. We practice faith, courage, and hope as we encounter life unfolding one day at a time. Honesty and willingness are among the tools we use to face and live life successfully. We develop patience and perseverance, being aware of the power our thoughts have in determining how our day goes. We experience freedom when we remain accountable for our behavior and atone for any of our actions that harm others. We trust the connection we are building with a power greater than ourselves as we reach out in service.

We cannot share what we do not have. The quality of our recovery will be what attracts the suffering addict to Pills Anonymous and to our newfound way of living. If rejected, we are careful not to force the newcomer or prospective member to accept our program. We let go on a positive note and leave the door open. Those with a change of heart are less hesitant to return when their first encounter was open and welcoming. We are wise to practice patience, compassion, unconditional love, and unequivocal acceptance.

The principles we embraced while working the steps include, but are not limited to, open-mindedness, surrender, hope, faith, trust, courage, honesty, humility, willingness, integrity, forgiveness, patience, acceptance, sincerity, discipline, vigilance, and persistence. We make an effort to put these principles in motion as we go through our day. With practice, they become part of who we are. Adherence to the spiritual principles of the Twelve Steps fosters an integrity that becomes as natural as breathing. We find that these principles will come to our aid in all situations. Encounters with family, co-workers, and everyone else outside the rooms of Pills Anonymous are all opportunities to live the principles of our recovery. We have found that it does not benefit us to be selective when choosing which steps or principles to apply in our lives. Our experience shows that only practicing Steps One and Twelve will not keep us clean or nurture our emotional growth. We must practice all of the steps and all the principles in our daily lives. It is a recipe that has worked for many. We have come to know that not using is the most important thing in our lives, yet by itself, this is not enough. We also want to be happy, to know joy, and to be free. For this, we must walk the path of recovery, using the tools we have picked up along the way, receiving support by holding the hands of those in the rooms of Pills Anonymous, and giving support by holding our hands out to the still suffering pill addict.

Filled with gratitude, we walk lightly in the world, unburdened, with our heads up and our hearts open. Conducting our lives in this way carries a message of hope to all who may cross our path. At times, we may not need to say a word. Simply living by example, we can attract the weary addict. Just as someone was there for us, we must have our hands out with an understanding only a fellow sufferer can know.

OUR MEMBERS' EXPERIENCE
WITH STEP TWELVE

ONE LEAF AT A TIME

I had done my first eleven steps. All that remained was the Twelfth. I was completely unaware of my spiritual transformation. I was sharing my story at the treatment facility I had attended only a year earlier, and I said, "I am the same person I was last year." My friends from my home group who supported me by coming to hear me speak told me otherwise! They said I was not the same person. I was no longer the miserable, self-loathing chap I used to be.

You see, I hadn't had a burning bush experience. Instead, my Higher Power seemed to reach down with His holy lighter and set each leaf on fire, one at a time, extinguishing one before lighting the next. If I looked at yesterday, I could see no change, but if I looked back over a period of months, I could see the transformation. It truly was an awakening.

I was scared. This meant I might now be expected to sponsor someone. What if I did something wrong? What if...if I said something that killed someone?! I really thought that way. I actually thought I had that much power—or was it lack of power...or lack of confidence? My Higher Power, God as I call him/her, took care of me. I didn't know that at the time. As it turned out, nobody asked me to sponsor them for quite some time, and when they did, it was just to satisfy their counselor in rehab. The first people I sponsored never called me after they got out of rehab. I felt bad for them, but I stayed clean. I might not be the greatest sponsor. I haven't been able to help any sponsees past the Ninth Step. Facing the reality of making those amends just seems to put the brakes on recovery for some people, even if that is the step where I think our program really starts to work.

The Twelfth Step for me is not just about being a sponsor. There are so many other ways to carry the message. I'm amazed when a newcomer in rehab says, "Thank you for bringing this meeting in here." Don't they know that this is another way of carrying the message—and that it keeps me clean? If you ever get a chance to go to a meeting in a hospital or prison, go! It will blow you away!

I have been told by more than one person that it really makes a difference to them when they see me at meetings.

Going to meetings regularly is another way we carry the message. Simply sharing my experience, strength, and hope during a meeting can really hit home to a newcomer or even a long-term member who gets something from my share. It feels good for me to let go of things at a meeting, but at the same time, when I do share what's happening with me, I am also carrying the message. Leading off a meeting by sharing for ten minutes about how it was, what happened, and how it is today may be just what someone needs to hear. I remember after a meeting a fellow came up to me and said he really identified with me and what I said—because we were born in the same town. You never know what might turn someone's head; you just never know.

Talking after the meeting, while standing outside the meeting place or over coffee or a meal with a bunch of pill addicts, can make a difference to someone. There was a time earlier in my recovery when I was asked repeatedly to go out after meetings for a bite to eat and some fellowship, but I was too busy. Didn't they know who I thought I was? One day, after a meeting, I kept missing turns to my house and ended up at the restaurant the group went to. I had the time of my life, and right there and then, I began to belong. To this day, I still go out after my home group meeting for a bite to eat. It's just a regular part of the plan, and everyone is welcome. We usually have a group of a dozen or so and we talk about anything and everything. As we get to know each other this way, many a person has found out that even though we have different jobs and backgrounds, we do have similarities and we do belong. This is Twelfth Step work.

I had the opportunity to go to the first P.A. conference in Las Vegas and the second one in Tempe. I got to crawl right inside this fellowship and participate in the beginnings of P.A. as a worldwide organization. Together we were there, together we participated. Having had a spiritual awakening as the result of these steps, we tried to carry this message to other pill addicts—all over this world—and to practice these principles in all our affairs. Spending those days in fellowship helped me stay clean—and I hope that's working the Twelfth Step, too!

Regularly doing our maintenance steps—Ten, Eleven, and Twelve—actually helps to make practicing and living these principles in all our affairs almost effortless. I am powerless, not only over my addiction, but over almost everything in my life. There is a power greater than me that will make things right, in spite of myself. If I take a regular inventory of how I am behaving, and quickly make amends, then my connection to that Higher Power is maintained. We remain buddies and everything works out. Someone once said, "In the end, everything works out. If it's not right, then it's not the end!"

I had a counselor in rehab who used to say, "Everyone is here to show an example—some to show a good one and some to show a bad one. You learn from both." I think that's interesting and true. I hope my examples are good, but even if I really screw up, someone will still learn from me.

ALIVE AND CONNECTED

When I embarked on my journey of recovery, I simply could not imagine that I would ever have anything to offer another person, let alone another pill addict who needed help. I felt so messed up! In the ending stages of my using, my addiction to pills had stripped me of my humanity. This sounds rather drastic as I write it on paper today, but it really is the complete truth. I was filled with guilt, shame, and remorse, and suffered from debilitating anxiety and depression. Other than those feelings, I was devoid of any real emotion. I no longer laughed, cried, or connected with anyone on an emotional level. I was utterly alone in the world and had absolutely no hope that it could ever get better.

After a few months of stringing together some clean days and starting on the steps with my sponsor, I began to feel better, more human. Even so, Step Twelve seemed like some far-away land that only other people would get to visit. How very wrong I was. I see now what I couldn't yet see at that time. I had to take each step one at a time, in order. When I did, my spirit began to awaken, and with each passing day I became more alive, more connected to both my Higher Power and the people around me. I cleaned house by doing a searching and fearless moral inventory. I shared my amends list with my sponsor and held nothing back. I cleaned my side of the street by doing each of my amends with purpose and without delay. I continued to take inventory. I prayed and meditated—a lot! By doing all of these things and taking the suggestions of my sponsor, I was able to get down to the causes and conditions that had been troubling me my whole life. There were so many things inside of me that I was blind to, buried under all of the drugs and bad behavior, until I worked the steps.

What a revelation that was for me! By following the steps in this way, I was more than ready for Step Twelve when I reached it. Sometimes I would feel a little nervous when talking to a newcomer and I would worry in advance that I would say the wrong thing or not be able to come up with an answer. I realize now that this was my character defect of perfectionism at its worst. I find that if I rely on my Higher Power's help, our literature, and an honest sharing of my own experience, strength, and hope, then the right words come to me. I have also come to understand that nothing I say or don't say will keep another person clean. My job is to carry the message, and when I carry out that task to the best of my ability, my own recovery is strengthened.

Practicing the principles of our program in all areas of my life is what carries me through each day with peace and serenity. No matter what I am experiencing, I rely on the

Twelve Steps as my guide. If I am feeling irritable, grouchy, sad, or tired, I ask myself a series of questions that help me figure out what's going on. Did I pray and meditate today? Am I harboring a resentment against someone that needs to be addressed? Do I owe an amends? Am I trying to control the outcome of something that needs to be turned over to my Higher Power? I almost always find relief by looking at my daily life in this manner. If the answer is still unclear or my thinking feels muddled, I reach out to another person by talking with my sponsor or participating in a meeting. At other times, the best medicine is to work with a sponsee or newcomer. By getting out of myself, I let go of the old, selfish behavior which has proven many times to be my downfall. I cannot feel anger, resentment, or fear unless I am thinking about myself.

Today I truly enjoy carrying the message by being of service and I like to keep my program fresh by finding new ways to do this. Whether it is answering the phone or pouring coffee, I can stay connected to the fellowship that saved my life, and practice Step Twelve at the same time. Steps One through Eleven teach me how to live life clean. Step Twelve encourages me to teach someone else how truly awesome recovery can be, and for all of this, I will be forever grateful to P.A. and the Twelve Steps of recovery!

WORKING STEP TWELVE

Like Steps Ten and Eleven, Step Twelve is a maintenance step, one that keeps us from returning to our active addiction. We may have experienced a spiritual awakening as a result of working the Twelve Steps, but we can always go back to sleep. Carrying the message of recovery to other addicts and practicing the spiritual principles of recovery in all our affairs is our best bet if we want to continue being happy, joyous, and free. Writing our answers to these questions, and discussing them with our sponsor can help us understand the importance of practicing the Twelfth Step.

1. What has my spiritual awakening been like as a result of working the steps?

2. How is my life different today as a result of working the steps?

3. In what ways has my spiritual awakening been a process, an event, or both?

4. What is the message that the Twelfth Step refers to, and in what ways was this message carried to me?

5. Why and how has Pills Anonymous been able to reach me in a way no one else could?

6. Why is it important to carry the message by sharing our experience, strength, and hope, rather than by giving advice?

7. What are some of the different ways in which we can carry the message?

8. What am I currently doing to carry the message?

9. In what ways am I being of service to others in Pills Anonymous? How am I being of service outside of Pills Anonymous?

10. How can I do more to carry the message? What is preventing me from expanding this area of my life?

11. How does it make me feel when I carry the message? Why do we say, "We keep what we have by giving it away"?

12. What are my expectations about the outcome of my service? Is my service unconditional?

13. What is my understanding of sponsorship? How well do I carry the message of recovery through sponsorship? What can I learn from the people I sponsor?

14. What are the spiritual principles I have learned in working the Steps?

15. What have I learned about the value of the principles that I can practice in all my affairs? Explain how these spiritual principles apply to each step: honesty (Step One), hope and openness (Step Two), willingness and faith (Step Three), courage and integrity (Steps Four and Five), willingness (Step Six), humility (Step Seven), self-discipline and love for others (Steps Eight and Nine), perseverance (Step Ten), spiritual awareness (Step Eleven), and service (Step Twelve).

16. How can I practice these principles in my daily life and in all my relationships?

17. Which of these spiritual principles are the most challenging for me today?

18. In what areas of my life have I found it most difficult to practice these principles?

19. What tools can I use to make sure I practice these principles even when I do not feel like it?

20. In reflecting on where I have come from and where I am today, how important has this program been in changing my life? In what ways can I express my gratitude today?

21. What is the message I am living, and what will I leave for the suffering addicts who come to this program after I am gone?

THE TWELVE TRADITIONS OF PILLS ANONYMOUS

1. Our common welfare should come first; personal recovery depends upon P.A. unity.

2. For our group purpose there is but one ultimate authority—a loving God as He may express Himself in our group conscience. Our leaders are but trusted servants; they do not govern.

3. The only requirement for membership is a desire to stop using pills.

4. Each group should be autonomous, except in matters affecting other groups or P.A. as a whole.

5. Each group has but one primary purpose—to carry its message to the addict who still suffers.

6. A P.A. group ought never endorse, finance or lend the P.A. name to any related facility or outside enterprise, lest problems of money, property or prestige divert us from our primary purpose.

7. Every P.A. group ought to be fully self-supporting, declining outside contributions.

8. Pills Anonymous should remain forever nonprofessional, but our service centers may employ special workers.

9. P.A., as such, ought never be organized, but we may create service boards or committees directly responsible to those they serve.

10. Pills Anonymous has no opinion on outside issues; hence the P.A. name ought never be drawn into public controversy.

11. Our public relations policy is based on attraction rather than promotion; we need always maintain personal anonymity at the level of press, radio, television and films.

12. Anonymity is the spiritual foundation of all our Traditions, ever reminding us to place principles before personalities.

The Twelve Traditions of
Pills Anonymous
Introduction

There is a tendency among newer Pills Anonymous members to think that the Twelve Steps are more important than the Twelve Traditions. In meetings we sometimes hear, "Work the steps or die," or "What step are you working on right now?" We do not usually hear the same emphasis placed on learning and using the Twelve Traditions. The Twelve Steps are, after all, the keys to our personal recovery, and that is clearly our main focus when we first come into the program. As newcomers, we rarely stopped to think what our personal recovery would have been like if the groups we regularly attended had been torn apart by internal controversy. We took it for granted that the groups existed, and that there were meetings for us to attend. But when our self-centered fog begins to clear we realize our personal recovery depends on the health of our groups, and that the health of our groups depends on how well our members understand and apply the Twelve Traditions. No group is forced to follow the traditions, but in our experience, groups that embrace the traditions tend to flourish, and so do their members.

Another saying frequently heard in our rooms is, "We keep what we have by giving it away." Once we begin to develop some empathy for others by working Steps Four through Nine, and we experience even a glimmer of the spiritual awakening described in Step Twelve, we start wanting to transcend our habitual selfishness by helping others, especially those who suffer from the disease of pill addiction. We are being of service to other pill addicts just by attending meetings, but with the encouragement of our sponsors, many of us take on more service within our fellowship. We help set up and clean up the meeting space, make coffee, greet newcomers, and participate in group business meetings. We may take on the responsibility of serving as the group's secretary or treasurer, or as its representative at larger service meetings. When we get involved in service work of any kind, we usually discover that other members may have a variety of ideas about how to render a particular service, and that these ideas sometimes differ from our own. The Twelve Traditions teach us how to work together in harmony to achieve our common goal of carrying the message of recovery to the pill addict who still suffers. As we learn how vital service is for our recovery, we look to the traditions to guide our efforts, and we come to understand how essential our traditions are to our personal recovery.

The Twelve Traditions were written as guidelines for twelve-step organizations. In most cases they cannot be directly applied to other organizations that have different structures and goals. However, we soon learn that the spiritual principles of our Twelve Traditions can be of great value when we use them in our own lives. Acceptance, anonymity, commitment, compassion, courage, faith, fidelity, freedom, gratitude, harmony, humility, integrity, love, prudence, responsibility, selflessness, service, simplicity, surrender, trust, tolerance, unity, and willingness are some of the spiritual principles that guide us. These principles can become personal standards of conduct. By studying, applying, and practicing them, we vastly enrich our own lives and the lives of those around us.

Tradition One

"Our common welfare should come first; personal recovery depends upon P.A. unity."

Nothing is more important in P.A. than our groups. We often say that newcomers are the most important people in our rooms, but we must also realize that the group as a whole is more important than the newcomer. Without our groups and the meetings they hold, the newcomer would have nowhere to go. We depend on the support of our fellow pill addicts, so without meetings, it would be far more difficult for most of us to sustain our personal recovery. Without meetings to attend, many pill addicts would surely die from the disease of pill addiction. The Twelve Steps of Pills Anonymous are guidelines we follow as individuals to recover from our addiction to pills, and the Twelve Traditions are guidelines we follow to preserve our Pills Anonymous groups.

The importance of our common welfare cannot be overstated. By keeping the First Tradition uppermost in our minds, we give ourselves and pill addicts who still suffer a fighting chance to recover. In our experience, individual pill addicts on their own have little chance to stop using pills and put their disease into remission. Feeling isolated and friendless, most of us could not bear the guilt, depression, and desperation we faced when we were confronted with the wreckage we were causing. When we had to deal with disappointed parents, spouses, friends, and employers, or with the financial or legal problems we brought upon ourselves, we sought refuge in blame and self-pity, and retreated into loneliness and despair. Some of us tried to find solutions in religion or psychiatry, but despite our best efforts, we could not stop using pills. Finally, in desperation, we sought the help of others in Pills Anonymous, and began to experience the astounding therapeutic value of one pill addict helping another. What we had completely failed to accomplish alone became a real possibility when we began to accept the help of other people just like us.

Imagine what our lives might be like today if, after finally mustering the courage to attend a meeting, we had walked into a squabbling, dysfunctional P.A. group full of hostility, disagreement, and mistrust. Instead, we were welcomed with sincere love, affection, and acceptance. We were warmly embraced and enthusiastically encouraged to keep coming back. Members offered their time and attention to unconditionally help us. As newcomers, we were astonished that these people seemed to be able to live normal lives without the use of pills. They also seemed to possess what we could never imagine having ourselves—confidence and serenity. If disturbances or conflicts had disrupted the harmonious atmosphere of those first meetings, we might have never come back.

We also came to understand that without the support and encouragement of our fellow pill addicts, sustaining our individual programs of recovery would not be possible. Our determined commitment to the spiritual principle of unity stems from the simple fact that we need other recovering pill addicts in order for the Twelve Steps to work. We need sponsors to guide us through the steps, and we need to sponsor others. We need to attend meetings. Attending meetings energizes our personal rehabilitation by fostering the growth and development of a spiritual immune system that protects us from relapse. Without our meetings, we have found that we become more susceptible to the disease of pill addiction and its attendant miseries. Without unity, our meetings would not be an effective weapon in our daily battle against this disease.

Unity does not mean uniformity. We are not governed by our leaders or forced to conduct our recovery program in any particular way. We do not require conformity from our members. Instead, we celebrate our individuality and the diversity of our fellowship, encouraging personal freedom of thought, belief, expression, and action. At the same time, with so few constraints and so much freedom, we have a responsibility to avoid saying or doing anything that might endanger the group or the fellowship as a whole. It is because of the group that we were able to escape from the bondage of pill addiction and enjoy a satisfying new way of life. Endangering the unity of our groups jeopardizes the freedom and happiness of all our members, and threatens to extinguish the bright ray of hope P.A. offers to those still suffering from the disease.

If we accept the idea that unity is essential to the preservation of Pills Anonymous, we must ask ourselves what we can do to put this spiritual principle into practice. We can begin by treating each other with kindness. Our love and respect for each other helps fellow members feel comfortable and safe, and attracts newcomers who strengthen us all, fueling our sense of common purpose. As we work the steps, our self-centeredness diminishes and we find our communication skills improving. We learn to become active listeners, actually hearing what others have to say and empathizing with their feelings. We learn to express our own opinion without arrogance or fear of reprisal, and we become capable of disagreeing without being disagreeable. As we grow, we find that we no longer need to be right all the time, and when things do not go our way, we can simply "let go and let God."

Unity begins with humility. When we are humble, understanding our true position in relation to God and our fellow man, conflict seems to melt away. As our perspective improves, we find it easier to render selfless service to our fellowship. We attend meetings regularly, greet people at the door, make coffee, and share honestly and responsibly. We volunteer to be on committees and take service positions at the group, area, region, or world levels. In all these activities we try to remember our primary purpose, which is to carry our message of recovery to the pill addict who still suffers. To carry this message effectively, we must place our common welfare above all else.

Unity is essential to the survival of the individual pill addict, the P.A. group, and P.A. as a whole. With unity as a guiding principle, no disagreement or problem is ever more important than our need for each other's support. We come to understand and accept that the common welfare of Pills Anonymous must always come first, and that with faith in our Higher Power, we can find the strength to overcome differences and work together toward our shared goal of recovery.

Our Members' Experience with Tradition One

I Am So Grateful

Since I was blessed with the gift of recovery, I have gone to a lot of meetings. I took the "ninety meetings in ninety days" recommendation seriously, and I easily averaged one meeting per day during my first year. I still try to make it to five or six meetings per week, because I am reminded by almost every relapse story I hear that it started with not going to meetings.

The first time I attended a twelve-step meeting, I felt like I was home, that I belonged. I have attended meetings of other fellowships and I can find lots of similarities, but nothing compares with being in a P.A. meeting and hearing someone share something that reminds me, "Oh, yeah, I did that," and then the healing thought, "Wow, I *am* powerless over this disease." This has happened often, and I hear it from lots of newcomers. Our fellowship is a blessing, and I am so grateful that it was available for me when I got out of treatment.

I have taken on various service commitments at different levels, and our First Tradition has guided me through each experience. We all have differences of opinion on how things should be done and, as a pill addict sometimes I think I know what's best for everyone else. That is selfish, self-centered behavior. When I think that way, I need to get back to my Higher Power. I do not always know what's best for me, let alone anyone else. This tradition tells me I need to try to do what is best for the P.A. group, not necessarily what makes me or other individuals feel better.

I believe that if our common welfare didn't come first, P.A. groups would be splitting up into different factions with their own ways of doing things. When I first heard the Twenty Questions reading at the beginning of our meetings, I hated it. The questions made me very uncomfortable and I didn't understand why we read them. Now I love those questions and I believe they are a valuable tool for the newcomer. Most of us can answer "yes" to almost all of them, but what if I had tried to impose my selfish feelings on the group, and somehow I was able to sway the group to stop reading them? How many newcomers would then miss the opportunity to hear the questions and to give serious thought to their behavior and to why they were at a P.A. meeting? That was what made me uncomfortable, but ultimately helped me to better understand my addiction, and to feel like I belonged here.

WORKING TRADITION ONE

We can perhaps best understand Tradition One by examining our own behavior. We have a tendency to become experts on the First Tradition when someone else seems to be disregarding it, but as we have learned from working the Twelve Steps, keeping the focus on ourselves and on our own behavior helps us to progress on the path of recovery. Here are some questions that might help us to improve our understanding of Tradition One and the ways in which we can put it into practice.

1. Do I sometimes gossip about individual members in my group or in the fellowship? How does this affect me, the people I am gossiping with, and the people we are talking about?

2. How do I respond when someone says something that rubs me the wrong way?

3. Am I sometimes argumentative or contentious with other members? How does this affect the unity of our group, service work, or fellowship?

4. What do I do when there is a conflict between myself and another member, or between myself and an entire group? How do my actions serve to either divide us or bring us together? How do I make sure that the unity of the fellowship comes first in these situations?

5. In what ways am I judgmental of the behavior of other members, taking their inventory instead of my own?

6. Have I criticized other P.A. groups, or made comparisons between "my" meeting and other meetings? What effect does this have on our common welfare?

7. How do I further my sense of belonging to my group and P.A. as a whole? For example, do I attend and share in meetings regularly, greet newcomers, set up

chairs, clean up after the meeting, or make myself available as a sponsor?

8. How frequently do I reinforce my commitment to Pills Anonymous and strengthen my ties to the group by taking on other service positions, such as chairperson, treasurer, or general service representative? Why is this important?

9. Have I decided whether or not to take on any service position because of the people I would be working with? Have I sought out service positions so I could work with members I like? Have I avoided or left positions that required me to work with members I do not care for? Why is it so important to "place principles before personalities"?

10. In what ways do I try to increase my knowledge about P.A. as a whole, including the functions of P.A. World Services?

11. How can I apply some of the spiritual principles of Tradition One—unity, humility, surrender, acceptance, selflessness, love, anonymity, and commitment—in my role as a P.A. member and in my daily life?

TRADITION TWO

"For our group purpose there is but one ultimate authority—a loving God as He may express Himself in our group conscience. Our leaders are but trusted servants; they do not govern."

Our Twelfth Step suggests that we carry the message of recovery to other pill addicts, and we have found that one of the best ways to do that is to form groups in which we share our experience, strength, and hope with each other. When we form a group, which is a meeting of two or more pill addicts, we soon find that opportunities for service arise. There is a need for someone to arrange for the meeting place, someone to run the meeting, someone to provide coffee or refreshments, someone to welcome the newcomer, someone to make sure there is literature, and so forth. Each group has but one primary purpose—to carry the message to the pill addict who still suffers—but who decides exactly what needs to be done, and who decides the best way to do it?

There are many problems that arise when people, even those who do not have the disease of pill addiction, come together and form a group. There may be differences of opinion, power struggles, and hurt feelings that threaten to tear the group apart. For pill addicts, whose disease is characterized by extreme self-absorption and lack of consideration for others, these pitfalls might be hard to avoid. Pill addicts are also prone to rebellion against authority, and many of us would be reluctant to participate in this program if we were forced to follow the dictates of an individual, or even a group or committee.

So who runs P.A.? This is a question many of us asked when we entered these rooms. As pill addicts we tried to control people and things, and manipulate them to our advantage, so as newcomers to Pills Anonymous, many of us naturally assumed there must be one person, or perhaps a committee, that was in charge of the program. Nothing could be farther from the truth.

We learned in Step One that we were powerless and could not manage our own lives. In Step Two we came to believe that a power greater than ourselves could restore us to sanity, and in Step Three we turned our will and our lives over to the care of a Higher Power, whom many of us choose to call God. As individuals working the Twelve Steps, we are learning to surrender to a power greater than ourselves, and as groups we must learn to do exactly the same thing. At the suggestion of Tradition Two, we strive to always invite a loving God to be in charge of our groups, and we pray only for knowledge of His will for the group and for the power to carry that out.

The mechanism for making God the ultimate authority in our fellowship is called a group conscience. When we stop using pills and begin working the Twelve Steps, we gradually become aware of our self-centered behavior and its effect on others. Our conscience is reawakened. Similarly, when recovering pill addicts come together in groups and practice the Twelve Traditions, we develop a collective conscience. When we consult that collective conscience regularly, we allow God to shape the decisions and actions of our groups, as well as the fellowship as a whole. Our success in relying on a group conscience to guide our affairs largely depends on our willingness as individuals to seek direction from a Higher Power. When we bring that willingness into the group setting, we invite a spiritual presence into our meetings, activities, and service committees.

Surrendering to the group conscience begins with the principle of anonymity. A true group conscience based on this spiritual principle means that all members are treated as equals, regardless of clean date, experience, or background. No one member or group has a monopoly on the knowledge of a Higher Power's will. When issues or problems arise, all members are encouraged to share their ideas and solutions, and the other members are encouraged to listen with open minds. We learn to ask, "*What* is right?" instead of, "*Who* is right?" When all the points of view have been presented and heard, solutions often become apparent and there will be a unanimous consensus on what to do. At other times, it might be necessary to take a vote in order to make a decision. After the votes are tallied, we apply the spiritual principles of our steps and traditions, and learn to gracefully accept the consensus of the group even if we disagree with the majority.

Group decisions are never written in stone. Just as our understanding of our Higher Power's will for us changes as we proceed through the process of recovery, so does the conscience of the group, which can change as a result of time and circumstance. "We've always done it that way," or "We voted on that last month," are insufficient reasons for suppressing a call for change. We must remain flexible and open-minded so that we are always in a position to follow the will of our Higher Power.

After a group has sought direction from a loving God, it may ask some of its members to carry out its policies. The group may create various service positions, such as chairperson, literature coordinator, greeter, coffee maker, secretary, treasurer, or service representative (one who represents the group at meetings consisting of other P.A. groups). The group may elect or appoint members to carry out these tasks, but these members are not considered special in any way. Although they sometimes must exercise leadership in their respective positions, we refer to them as trusted servants because we trust them to serve, care for, and represent the needs of the group.

This trust is mutual. As a group we have faith that the members we select to serve will carry out their duties responsibly—by applying spiritual principles, acting with our common welfare in mind, and always seeking to further our primary purpose. We support them and help them in any way we can. In turn, our trusted servants are responsible to the group and to the loving Higher Power who has expressed Himself through the group conscience. Our trusted servants serve us best when they do not govern, but lead by personal example. They are honest and open, do not seek praise or special treatment, and remain humble and teachable, cultivating and expanding their knowledge of all aspects of service. They avoid seeking prestige or control, and try to limit the amount of time they stay in any one service position, so that other pill addicts can experience the rewards of service work.

Service to the fellowship of Pills Anonymous is indeed handsomely rewarded—not with money or fame, but with personal growth. We develop a better relationship with the God of our understanding, and we also learn how to get along better with our fellow human beings. We begin to enjoy the limitless freedom that comes from letting go of our innate desire for control, leaving that responsibility entirely in the supremely capable hands of our Higher Power.

OUR MEMBERS' EXPERIENCE WITH TRADITION TWO

IT'S HOW WE MAKE ALL OUR DECISIONS

I never paid much attention to the traditions until I began to get involved in service at the group level. I regularly attended a meeting for a few months and developed plenty of opinions about how the meeting wasn't being run correctly. The chairs weren't set up properly, the right readings weren't being used, the format was wrong, the food was unhealthy, and the people chosen to chair the meeting didn't have a good message. But the final straw was watching two treasurers in a row waltz off with the group's money. I complained bitterly to my sponsor about all this, and after he stopped laughing, he suggested that I attend the group's next business meeting and voice my opinions. I took his suggestion.

That was my first business meeting and my first experience with a group conscience. At the conclusion, I walked away with the treasurer's job. Today I can honestly say that until I began to regularly attend the business meetings and share responsibility for what was going on, I was not a part of that group. It was through service to the group that I stopped living in the "me" and started experiencing the "we" of this program.

My biggest challenge in the business meetings was that I knew too much. I had owned my own business and had served on the boards of various non-profit organizations for many years, so I thought I knew how meetings should be run—and I certainly didn't see God being a part of it. Fortunately, we had a few members with significant clean time and a strong understanding of the traditions to guide us. Every business meeting began with a simple prayer—often the Serenity Prayer. Sometimes a member would pray that we act selflessly, reaffirming that our common welfare and unity should come first and that our primary purpose was to carry the message to the addict who still suffers. These guiding principles seemed to help all of us practice selflessness. While having an understanding of the other traditions is crucial to help guide our group, I believe the Second Tradition is the one that comes into play every time we meet—it's how we make all our decisions.

We didn't have a lot of money coming into our group, and at our business meetings we'd have to decide how to allocate our meager resources. Once we paid the rent for our meeting space, we had to decide what literature, clean-time chips, and meeting refreshments to buy, and how much we should donate to the larger service body. I had never really considered these questions before, and there was much more to consider than I had initially thought. I didn't even know what literature we had or the cost of our rent! I got a dose of humility when I began to realize how little I knew. Despite that, in the beginning, I urgently wanted people to adopt my opinions. Thank God for the old-timers though, who demonstrated patience and understanding, setting aside their own opinions, asking other people what they thought, and encouraging minority opinions to be fully aired. I eventually saw how I was being self-centered and selfish, trying to have things my way again. I began to understand the meaning of being a trusted servant and the need to "let go and let God."

It was through my understanding of the Second Step that I came to understand how God "expresses Himself in our group conscience," as the Second Tradition says. My first experience with a power greater than myself that could restore me to sanity was the P.A. group itself. When I attended a meeting and listened to other recovering pill addicts, I saw myself in their stories, heard messages of recovery that seemed to be meant for me, found solutions to my problems that had escaped me, and gained hope that I otherwise lacked. Even though I was suspicious of the idea of *God*, I could readily believe that a spirit greater than all of us was moving through the meeting. I could even feel that power within me when I honestly shared from my own experience and delivered a message of hope and freedom from active addiction. I clearly believed that the meeting carried a power that was greater than the sum of its participating pill-addict parts.

I have found that our business meetings can work the same way, if we hold to our primary purpose and practice the principles of the program. I have found that I can never predict who God will be speaking through on any given subject. It often has nothing to do with the amount of time people have been clean. So, while I express my point of view, I also try to hold on a little less tightly to my precious opinions and remember to treat everyone with respect. Anyone can be God's messenger. A member I know with many years clean says that through the Second Tradition a group of addicts gathered to seek a spiritual solution to their common problem become a conduit for the word of God.

My sponsor told me early on that having a home group and a service commitment would help ensure my recovery. I believe I never would have relapsed if I had held to this formula. When I stopped going to meetings and being involved with other addicts seeking recovery, I fell back into selfishness, and I eventually began using again. I have seen this ethic of commitment to service demonstrated over and over by people with significant clean time. Since my first commitment as treasurer, I have gone on to serve as secretary, group representative, and greeter (my favorite so far). These commitments and being a part of my group's conscience at business meetings are what make me a responsible member of my home group. It makes *me* a part of the *we*.

WORKING TRADITION TWO

Understanding and practicing our Second Tradition is critical to the survival of Pills Anonymous. Many of us have discovered that service is also a critical component of our personal recovery. We must be vigilant about understanding and upholding the Second

Tradition if we want to continue as trusted servants in this fellowship. Honest reflection on these questions may encourage us to improve our service attitudes.

1. What resentments do I have against the leaders or the policies of any groups I have attended? Do I sometimes criticize the groups or their leaders? How does this affect me, the people I resent, the people I complain to, and the fellowship as a whole?

2. Why is it important for me to participate in my group's business meetings, and volunteer to be of help to the group in any capacity that is needed?

3. How does it affect my service when I seek credit and praise for the work I do in service?

4. What are some of my motivations for seeking or not seeking service positions?

5. Why is it a problem if I regard some service positions, like cleaning up after the meeting, as being less important than another position, such as secretary? How can I avoid the feeling that some chores are beneath me?

6. How does it affect me if I am reluctant to give up a service commitment because of the sense of control it gives me, or because of the prestige that goes with that position? How are my fellow pill addicts affected?

7. Am I ever afraid to voice my opinion in group business meetings because I think I will be ignored or contradicted? Why is this just as bad as trying to force my opinion on others?

8. In group discussions, what is my motivation if I sound off about matters on which I have no experience and little knowledge? How is this the same as being reluctant to speak because I feel like I have nothing to contribute?

9. What harm is there in believing that on certain matters my opinion is more important than someone else's?

10. Why is it so important to yield in good spirit to the group conscience and work cheerfully to support it?

Tradition Three

"The only requirement for membership is a desire to stop using pills."

Our own experience has taught us that a pill addict who does not want to stop will not stop. Lacking any desire to quit, we are doomed, but with even a tiny shred of willingness, conscious or unconscious, miracles can happen. Because of this, all we ask of our members is that they have a desire to stop using pills. The moment someone develops that spark of desire, no matter how small, they are qualified to become a member of Pills Anonymous. There are simply no other requirements for membership.

There is no way to measure a person's desire. The only one who truly knows what is in our heart is our Higher Power. Yet the act of walking into one of our meetings or talking to someone in the program is a sign of a pill addict's desire to change. Even a vague yearning to stop the cycle of pain that develops from pill addiction is enough to qualify someone as a member of Pills Anonymous. Membership in our fellowship is a personal decision that rests entirely in the hands of the individual, not the group. You are a pill addict when *you* say you are, and you are a Pills Anonymous member when *you* say so, whether you are still using pills or not.

Although membership is a personal decision, we can help pill addicts make that decision by warmly welcoming them into our fellowship, just as we were greeted when we washed up on these friendly shores. This is our chance to give back what was so freely given to us. We personally greet newcomers and introduce ourselves. We share our experience, strength, and hope with them before, during, and after meetings. We offer to exchange phone numbers, and above all, we encourage them to come back.

When we share our experience, we have to remember the broad inclusiveness of the wording of the First Step, in which we admit to being powerless over our addiction to, "pills and all other mind-altering substances." This includes alcohol, illegal drugs, and even some over-the-counter medications. At the same time, we understand that Pills Anonymous is a program of recovery for pill addicts. Although our addictions may not be limited to pills, most of us first came to P.A. because of our pill problems. If new members cannot identify with our message, they may feel they do not belong. Pill addiction is a deadly disease. Discouraging anyone, even inadvertently, from being a member of our group, may be a death sentence for that person.

In order to follow the Third Tradition, we must apply the spiritual principles of tolerance, compassion, humility, and anonymity. We go out of our way to be tolerant of those who do not think, act, or talk like us. We try to suspend our judgment and welcome everyone equally and unconditionally. We have learned from our predecessors that it is not a good idea to exclude anyone from membership because of their race, creed, color, religion, lack of religion, sexual preference, occupation, types of pills they used, socioeconomic status, smoking status, political beliefs, criminal history, level of education, or anything else that makes us seem different from each other. We do not care what anyone's favorite pill was, or how much or how little they used. Even if someone is still using pills, we encourage them to keep coming back. Exclusion of any kind, for any reason, risks the future of our organization, and consequently our own individual clean time.

We exercise our compassion by showing love and concern for all of our members, whether they are new in recovery or have accumulated many years of clean time. We demonstrate our humility when we remember that we are not God, and have no special power to judge another human being, no matter how long we have been in the program. We try to remain aware of our own shortcomings, and recall the fear and confusion we felt when we came to our first meeting. We refuse admission to no one, remembering, "There but for the grace of God, go I."

By remaining humble, which means we are no better or worse than anyone else, we embrace the principle of anonymity. Anonymity means more than simply guarding our identities from the public. Anonymity also means that no individual member or group is above any other, and that no one person is more important than the message we carry. Our program has no first- or second-class members, and we welcome everyone as equals. We are all equally subject to the devastation of the disease of pill addiction, and we all share an equal right to recovery.

Tradition Three conveys the blessing of freedom for those who practice it. We do not have to expend time and energy deciding who belongs and who does not. We do not have to figure out who needs our help and who does not. Instead, we are free to extend a loving, helping hand to anyone who wants what we have to offer.

OUR MEMBERS' EXPERIENCE WITH TRADITION THREE

DESIRE WAS THE ONLY THING I HAD

When I came into the world of recovery I had no idea what to expect. After thirteen very long and painful days in a detoxification facility, I entered a thirty-day drug and alcohol rehabilitation center. I had no understanding of what an addict was. In truth, I wasn't sure what I was—I just knew I wanted to be different. While in rehab, we were encouraged to attend twelve-step meetings and I gingerly tried a few here and there. I met some other pill addicts at the treatment center, and they were all a-buzz about Pills Anonymous. I was not ready to place myself into that niche because I was not done abusing pills. I attended a few meetings of another twelve-step program, but I was still not ready or willing to take any of their suggestions.

Not more than three months out of rehab I had a relapse. My relapse was not subtle or gentle; it was something pitiful and destructive. On my last day of drug abuse I was so frightened of what was happening to me that I ran to the nearest emergency room where I promptly (and very dramatically) fell apart. They quickly (and not so dramatically) transferred me to a psychiatric ward where I spent twenty-four hours being evaluated.

The next morning my husband showed up to sign me out and, much to my amazement, he was angry and said he didn't care what I did as long as I didn't do it around him or my daughter anymore. In essence, I was banned from home. During that long night and even longer ride home that morning, I contemplated my future. My husband graciously promised to provide for me, and said I could live anywhere I chose—just not at home with him. I could do whatever I wanted, but I wasn't going to drag my family through the pain anymore. "It's not because I don't love you," he said, "but I just can't watch you do this anymore." Do what? Live? This was how I knew to live. It felt dark and dreary, but it's what I knew—how to get to the next state of oblivion. I also knew that there were people out there like me who looked like they were happy.

My daughter was sent to live with my mother and father-in-law, so I was left with some time to plan my next step.

My first was to go to a Pills Anonymous meeting. I walked in late and everyone was laughing and having a good time. "They're laughing at you," my brain raced. "They know you're worthless and lost. They KNOW!" I needed a reality check! What they were doing was recovering and sharing. They were walking through their joys and sorrows together. They had what I wanted, and they let me come in. I was sincerely welcomed. I was introduced to everyone, particularly to other women. I was given the location of another meeting and I attended that one, too. In my haze of self-absorption I was asked to read preambles and traditions as part of the meeting format, but I had no idea how much the Third Tradition would really mean to me until months later.

When I went to meetings I was not always happy. In fact, I was usually unhappy, but I forced myself to keep going to meetings. My stubbornness had now become an asset. To every meeting, I took my pain and my drama. I arrived at meetings the way I was and they always let me in. Everyone said, "Keep coming back," and I thought it was personal praise. I thought I was so important that they wanted me to come back! Ego and all, I was always allowed in. The only requirement for membership was a desire to stop using pills. That was it, and I definitely met that criterion. Eventually, I arrived at meetings not with pain and drama, but with my happiness and my triumph over addiction.

I lived in a halfway house for women for nine months. The house had random drug tests and mandatory twelve-step meetings each day. At home with my husband, there were requirements I had to meet in order to be allowed to stay. Everywhere I looked, I felt like there were rules governing where I could go and what I could do—everywhere except Pills Anonymous. The only requirement there was my desire to stop using pills.

I passed a lot of judgment on others and, if it had been up to me alone, there were many people I would not have allowed into our fellowship. I wanted it all for myself—exclusive rights and membership! I wanted complete control. I believe this is why the Third Tradition exists. With people like me in charge, there would be no successful recovery from pill addiction. With people like me in charge, I would be the only member, and that would be very bad, indeed!

I am alive today in part because of the Third Tradition. My acceptance of the first three steps is essential for me to have faith in a power greater than myself, the power that I call my God. Acceptance and faith are at the core of my clean time, but it is the Third Tradition that allows people like me in the door and consistently welcomes us back. In the first days of my recovery, it seemed like an insurmountable requirement, but today I know that desire was the only thing I had for a while. Today I have deep gratitude for that succinctly laid-out tradition: The only requirement for membership is a desire to stop using pills.

WORKING TRADITION THREE

We may nod our heads in agreement as we read the Third Tradition, but putting it into practice is sometimes difficult. We all know how easy it is to slip into our old ways of thinking and evoke those old behaviors with which we used to be so comfortable. Many of us have found that unless we honestly appraise our actions on a regular basis, we may jeopardize our newfound freedoms, and perhaps even threaten our whole new pill-free way of life. By answering these questions, we can "take our temperature," and guard against the unwelcome recurrence of our disease.

1. Why is it important for me to resist the temptation to focus my attention on my friends in the fellowship rather than welcoming newcomers? What are some of the possible consequences of being inattentive to

some of our members, especially those who are new to the program?

2. How do I overcome my natural tendency to be less friendly to some members of my group because of their age, race, religion, or other perceived differences?

3. How can I avoid taking other members' inventories, holding them in higher or lower esteem because of my evaluation of their worth?

4. In what ways do I try to give each and every newcomer a warm and loving welcome, whether they are still using or not?

5. What is the potential risk of prejudging new members and saying to myself, "This person is going to make it," or "That person has no chance at all"?

6. When I talk to a newcomer or to members with less clean time than I have, how can I avoid setting myself up as an authority on Pills Anonymous? Why is it better to just honestly share my own experience, strength, and hope instead of trying to be an instructor?

7. Why is it important for me to invite new members along when going out for coffee after a meeting, or to other gatherings or activities that take place outside of meetings?

8. What are some of the things I can do to prevent myself from treating individual members differently because of their profession, fame, economic standing, social position, affiliations, or personal interests?

9. Are there any members I wish would not come to "my" meetings? What is wrong with avoiding some meetings because there are too many newcomers, or because my friends do not go there?

10. How can I apply Tradition Three to other areas of my life?

TRADITION FOUR

"Each group should be autonomous, except in matters affecting other groups or P.A. as a whole."

Just as Tradition Three defines individual membership in P.A., Tradition Four sets guidelines for P.A. groups. For individuals, the only requirement is a desire to stop using pills. For the group, the only requirement is that its actions do not adversely affect other groups or P.A. as a whole.

This policy of autonomy allows our groups the freedom to do almost anything they want in their effort to carry our message of recovery, as long as other groups and P.A. as a whole remain unaffected by their actions. Groups can meet whenever and wherever they wish, and can use any meeting format they choose. Meeting types vary widely. There are discussion meetings open to the public, closed meetings for pill addicts only, book-study meetings, speaker meetings, candlelight meetings, and so forth. Groups may also identify themselves as women's, men's, or LGBT meetings. P.A. groups can organize retreats and workshops, or have picnics, dances, campouts, and other social events to celebrate and carry the message of recovery. Every P.A. group is free to experiment and free to learn from such experimentation. Furthermore, any P.A. member may start a new P.A. group at any time.

Giving so much freedom to admittedly sick people such as ourselves might at first seem like a recipe for chaos and disaster. However, once we look carefully at the wording of Tradition Four, and think about what it means, we find that our options are, in fact, somewhat limited. The word "autonomy" comes from the Greek roots *auto* (self) and *nomos* (custom or law). Thus, "autonomy" means independence, or living by one's own laws. We could argue that one's own law could be that there are no laws, which of course would result in anarchy. Indeed, many of us have tried that approach to life, and we know first-hand that the consequences are misery and despair. The Pills Anonymous Steps and Traditions provide us with an attractive alternative. In the Third Step we individually "made a decision to turn our will and our lives over to the care of God as we understood Him." Similarly, in Tradition Two we acknowledge that, "for our group purpose there is but one ultimate authority—a loving God as He may express Himself in our group conscience." Therefore, our full understanding of the meaning of autonomy is that P.A. groups are independent, but are each governed by a Higher Power as expressed in the group conscience, and by the Twelve Steps and Twelve Traditions.

With freedom comes responsibility, so as groups we try to cultivate an attitude of respect for other groups and for P.A. as a whole. In the past, we were slaves to our pill addiction. We were impulsive and took little or no responsibility for our actions. Today, we think before we act. We soberly examine the consequences of our decisions, thoughtfully weighing their effect on ourselves and others. As individuals, we try to be honest about our motivation, listen to the suggestions of our sponsors, seek the wisdom of the Twelve Steps, and pray for knowledge of our Higher Power's will. As groups, we embrace the Second Tradition by surrendering to our Higher Power's will, and then examine our conduct in light of the other eleven Traditions.

For example, a group might want to decide which prayer to use in closing its meetings. Since each group's primary purpose is to carry the message to the pill addict who still suffers, we look first at how our decision will affect the newcomer. We examine the wording of the prayers, thinking about how the words might have sounded to us when we first entered the fellowship. We consider how they might sound to anyone new to the program.

We also ask if the prayer is closely identified with a particular religion, since it is possible that someone might think we are endorsing or expressing an opinion about that specific religion. Of course, no restrictions are placed on individual members, whose diversity we strongly encourage. Indeed, by avoiding direct or implied endorsements and opinions as a group, we allow the diversity of our individual members to flourish. In the end, after due consideration by the group, we choose a prayer that we believe best meets our group's needs and honors the P.A. Traditions.

Tradition Four guarantees each group the freedom of self-regulation, but being part of P.A. as a whole carries with it the responsibility to temper our independence with concern for other P.A. groups and regard for the entire fellowship. Achieving a balance between independence and responsibility is no easy task, and requires our reliance on a Higher Power, as well as adherence to the spiritual principles we have learned in our program.

One of our most important spiritual principles is unity. According to our First Tradition, our common welfare comes first, so we try to avoid doing anything that would foster divisiveness in our fellowship, either among our individual members, or between our groups. We demonstrate unity by handing out only Pills Anonymous Conference-approved literature in our meetings. Our individual members, of course, are free to read or use any literature they want on their own, but it is our responsibility as a group to carry the clear and undiluted message of Pills Anonymous in our meetings. One can easily imagine how quickly our fellowship would dissolve if each one of our groups chose their own smorgasbord of literature to distribute.

Unity goes hand in hand with the spiritual principle of anonymity. In this context, anonymity means that each group has an equal place in our fellowship, with equal rights and responsibilities. No group is more or less important than any other. We try not to praise or criticize other groups because of things like their size or the meeting format they use. We encourage a spirit of cooperation, not competition.

Another important spiritual principle is compassion. If a newcomer who is a man accidentally enters a women's meeting, our response should not be a harsh reprimand. Instead, we warmly welcome the new person and explain the difference between our meeting formats. We also provide some of our literature, some phone numbers of male members if possible, and a schedule of all our meetings. Whether the person can stay or has to leave is up to the group, but in either case we act with kindness and love. No matter what format our group uses, our primary purpose remains the same—to carry the message to the pill addict who still suffers.

We should also show our consideration for Pills Anonymous as a whole by maintaining the decorum of our group. It is critical that we always think about how our fellowship is viewed by society. We should treat our meeting facilities with respect, keeping them clean and in good order. We should act like good neighbors and responsible adults. Even the name a group chooses may reflect on P.A. as a whole. As soon as we identify ourselves in any way as members of Pills Anonymous, we become representatives of P.A. as a whole, and we should conduct ourselves in ways that positively reflect on our fellowship. If the public reputation of Pills Anonymous is somehow impaired, and prevents those in need from seeking recovery in our rooms, pill addicts may die.

OUR MEMBERS' EXPERIENCE
WITH TRADITION FOUR

A WAY THAT WORKS

It sometimes feels awkward for me to go into a meeting that is different from the ones I am used to. For example, some meetings read long opening statements, and I'm impatient for the readings to end and for the sharing to begin. Sometimes groups observe a moment of silence that seems to stretch into infinity. Sometimes I am irritated when there is "too much" laughter, and other times I want people to just lighten up. Some groups allow people to speak for a long time or more than once. No matter how these other meetings are run, my first thought is usually, "They're doing it all wrong!"

When I first came to recovery, I was so desperate for help that I paid little or no attention to how meetings were conducted, but as my time in recovery increased, I began to notice the differences. Soon, I became judgmental about how one meeting had too many readings, and that at another meeting people were loud and obnoxious, and so on. When I complained to my sponsor, she suggested that I read the Fourth Tradition.

What an eye-opener that was for me! I had to look up the word "autonomous," and found out it meant self-sufficiency, self-government, self-rule. In other words, any group could do anything it wanted! My pill-addict mind raced. I envisioned myself reinventing my home group, throwing out all the people I thought were losers, and getting everyone to do things "the right way." I had conveniently forgotten about the second part of the Fourth Tradition that says, "...except in matters affecting other groups or P.A. as a whole." I realized that we have to take into account other people, other groups, and P.A. as a whole! It seems that every time I fall in love with my own ideas, I also run up against the First Tradition, which reminds me that the most important thing is our unity. Our common welfare is more important than my own self-righteous demands.

I began to understand that Tradition Four allows each P.A. group the freedom to decide which meeting format to use, whether it will be an open or closed meeting, where to hold a meeting, how it would like to begin and end the meeting, and where to spend the funds collected at the meeting. At our business meetings, a group conscience is taken to decide what suits the needs of our particular group.

I also realized, though, that autonomy in P.A. does not mean that a group can change the wording of the Steps or Traditions to suit their taste. They shouldn't use or display outside literature at their meetings. Sticking to our steps and traditions and using only Conference-approved literature are practices essential to the strength and longevity of Pills Anonymous. I now understand that making these kinds of changes at the group level dilutes our message—and carrying the message is our primary purpose.

Personally, I wouldn't even want to attend a meeting in which changes to the P.A. Steps and Traditions had been made. I would not want to listen to a speaker who described a new cure for pill addiction that did not rely on the Twelve Steps of P.A. Our steps, traditions, and message of recovery are what got me clean, and what have allowed me to stay clean one day at a time. In my addiction, I tried many ways to quit using pills, none of which worked. In Pills Anonymous, I found a program that *does* work. For this once-suffering pill addict, that says it all!

That's why the message of recovery I try to pass on to other suffering pill addicts is based on our steps, traditions, and literature. Yes, my group can do whatever it wants, but if we interfere with other groups or P.A. as a whole, we get in the way of our P.A. unity and our primary purpose of helping those still suffering from this disease.

Working Tradition Four

The Fourth Tradition is extremely important to understand and practice. The survival of Pills Anonymous depends on this tradition, so both our personal recovery and the recovery of pill addicts still struggling with their disease are at stake. Taking personal and group inventories of how well we practice Tradition Four ensures that the ties that bind us together will always be stronger than the forces that could tear us apart. Answering these questions truthfully can help us grow spiritually and remain in harmony with the fellowship that has done so much for us.

1. How does my group make sure that its decisions do not adversely affect other P.A. groups or P.A. as a whole? How do we encourage our group members to always consider the Fourth Tradition before making decisions or taking action?

2. On what occasions have I been unfairly judgmental of a P.A. group by not respecting its right to do what it wants as long as other groups or P.A. as a whole are not affected?

3. Have I taken any groups' inventories (including my own), and held them in higher or lower esteem because of my evaluation? Has my home group also conducted itself in this way?

4. Are there times when I am overly insistent that I know the "right" way to do something? When visiting a new group, have there been times when I was irritated because they just did not do things the "right" way? What are some of the possible consequences of this type of thinking and behavior?

5. How does my group invite the presence of a Higher Power into its meetings, business meetings, special events, and social occasions?

6. Do my group and I think carefully and responsibly about our actions *before* we take them? How have my group and I applied the steps and traditions in making some of our recent decisions?

7. How do other members of my group and I share our knowledge of the P.A. Traditions with members who are not aware of them? Do we "preach from the pulpit" or simply share our experience, strength, and hope?

8. How do other members of my group and I demonstrate our compassion for the newcomer? In what ways do we go out of our way to welcome new people, make them feel comfortable, and do our best to keep them coming back?

9. How seriously do my group and I take the responsibility of making sure our meeting places are shown the utmost respect so that the image of P.A. will not be tarnished?

10. In what ways has my group been careless about how we conduct ourselves in public when we can be identified as members of Pills Anonymous? In what ways have I done this myself? What are some of the possible consequences we face for acting inappropriately?

11. How can I apply the principles of Tradition Four to other areas of my life, such as my family, school, job, or the clubs and organizations to which I belong?

TRADITION FIVE

"Each group has but one primary purpose — to carry its message to the addict who still suffers."

Our Fourth Tradition establishes guidelines for our groups to achieve their objectives, but does not say what those objectives should be. That information is presented here in Tradition Five, which clearly and concisely defines the single reason for the existence of every Pills Anonymous group and P.A. as a whole. The Fifth Tradition is a brief, simple summary of the aims and priorities of our fellowship. It is our mission statement.

The members of our fellowship have been given a special gift — the ability to help others escape from the slavery of addiction and find a new and meaningful way of life. The therapeutic value of one pill addict helping another is truly without parallel. We have seen time and again how pill addicts closely identify with other pill addicts, and are able to both give and receive recovery through the sharing of their experience, strength, and hope. Because our special ability to communicate with other pill addicts is the one thing we have to offer that few others can, it is the most important aspect of our fellowship. We attempt to do that one single thing really well.

We are careful to distinguish between our individual goals as recovering pill addicts and the goals of a Pills Anonymous group or P.A. as a whole. As individuals, we might to want to become good parents, strive to be successful in our careers, or spend our time helping others. We have the freedom to choose many different paths. We also have many different motives for attending a Pills Anonymous meeting. If we ask ourselves, "What's the main reason I'm here?" the answer might be, "To recover from my addiction to pills," or, "To get my court card signed," or, "So my wife will take me back." No matter why anyone is here, our fellowship says, "Just keep coming back." We encourage and celebrate the many reasons for which our members come to our meetings, but we do not support any such diversity of purpose for our groups.

The singleness of purpose expressed in Tradition Five, to carry the message to the pill addict who still suffers, prevents our groups from shifting their focus to other activities. We might turn our groups into social clubs, treatment facilities, or money-making enterprises, and while there is nothing wrong with such endeavors per se, these activities would distract us from carrying the message of recovery to pill addicts in distress, both inside and outside our rooms. As a result, pill addicts might die. Many of our own lives and the lives of those who have not yet found our fellowship depend on the clear and consistent message of hope and freedom carried by Pills Anonymous.

Nothing should divert a group from its primary purpose. Our members are encouraged to take personal responsibility for keeping our meetings recovery-oriented. We try to avoid distractions such as discussing group business or finances during meeting time, or socializing at the expense of helping another pill addict who may be in pain and need encouragement. When it comes to naming our group, choosing a meeting format, selecting our trusted servants, or establishing standards for group decorum, we rely on the Fifth Tradition for guidance. We regularly take a group inventory, and ask ourselves what we can do to improve our adherence to this tradition.

Step Twelve encourages us to carry the message of recovery to other pill addicts, for their benefit as well as ours. "We keep what we have by giving it away," is one of our most cherished sayings. Our experience in guiding others through the Twelve Steps has confirmed that the more we share our understanding of recovery with others, the more our own understanding increases. Tradition Five takes Step Twelve to the group level, and magnifies its effectiveness. We have seen that when an entire group comes together and focuses its energy on responsibly conveying the message of Pills Anonymous, the impact of the Twelfth Step is greatly multiplied, creating an atmosphere of recovery with a spiritual power that can accomplish miracles.

But what is our message? Simply put, it is that we can become free from active pill addiction. The message of hope we wish to carry to the pill addict who still suffers is that he or she can stop using pills, lose the all-consuming desire to take pills, and find a new way to live. The primary conduit for carrying this message is the Pills Anonymous meeting. In our meetings we try to share responsibly. We avoid long "pill-a-logs," which tend to convey the mess more than the message. Philosophy, religion, and politics are great topics for discussion, but not at a Pills Anonymous meeting. Instead, we share about how we got into recovery and how we have been able to stay clean through practicing the Twelve Steps. Sometimes we talk about the pain in our lives and how we are applying the steps to solve our problems without using. Sometimes we share the joy we experience as a result of practicing the spiritual principles of our program. In short, we stick to our primary purpose of carrying the message of recovery to the still-suffering pill addict. What we share can either further that purpose or detract from it. The choice is ours.

Because of the Fifth Tradition, our groups go to great lengths to make newcomers feel welcome. When new people arrive they may be terrified, angry, resentful, and lacking hope—yet we greet them warmly, as we ourselves would wish to be greeted. We reach out to them, comfort them, and love them until they can love themselves. We refrain from judging them or giving them advice. Instead, we empathize with them, remembering our own fears and doubts when we ventured into our first meeting. We share with them how our lives have changed because of Pills Anonymous.

The pill addict who still suffers may not be a newcomer. Many of us go through periods of doubt and desperation that challenge our recovery, no matter how long we have been clean. At times like this, our fellow pill addicts can help alleviate our suffering by carrying the message to us, regardless of how long they themselves have been in the program. Those of us who sponsor other pill addicts have experienced times when the people we sponsor were the ones carrying the message to us. This illustrates the precept of anonymity, which enables us to set our egos aside and place principles before personalities. The message of recovery can then freely circulate among all the members of our fellowship.

In addition to responsibly sharing in meetings, there are many other ways to carry the message of Pills Anonymous. When we engage in any type of service work, whether it is cleaning up after a meeting, being a sponsor, or representing our group at a World Service Conference, we are helping to bring recovery to pill addicts who still suffer. In fact, this is the real meaning of service in our fellowship. The goal of all service work is to help accomplish our primary purpose in one way or another.

Of course we may sometimes do service work to make ourselves feel more important, or to impress other pill addicts with our recovery. When these kinds of selfish motives arise, they may interfere with our ability to be of service to the fellowship. We can avoid such pitfalls by applying the spiritual principle of integrity. As individuals and as groups, we demonstrate our integrity by adhering to our principles, and when we are true to the principles embodied in the

Twelve Traditions, we are able to engage in proper service, doing the right thing for the right reasons.

Tradition Five is our program's lifeblood, and the key to our fellowship's unity. Our common goal binds our groups together in a strong and effective fellowship. As long as we remember that our primary purpose is to carry the message to pill addicts who still suffer, all will be well.

OUR MEMBERS' EXPERIENCE WITH TRADITION FIVE

HEY, THAT WAS *ME*!

Early in my search for recovery I struggled to stop using pills. I didn't want to use, but I kept doing it anyway. I would attend P.A. meetings and hold on to the hope that I could stop, because this group welcomed me with open arms. They did not criticize me, but loved and accepted me as a person who suffered from an addiction to pills. Outside the P.A. group I felt judged. When people saw I could not control my pill use, they said I had weak will, no self-discipline, poor moral fiber, or, as my own mom said, "You are too intelligent to do this." These attitudes just confirmed my own opinion that I was worthless and could not stop using.

The message I heard from P.A. was different. They said I could stop using pills if I just *wanted* to stop, and if I took some simple suggestions. Ironically, this message that kept me coming back was being delivered by people who also couldn't seem to help using pills, even though they didn't want to. They said that addiction was a disease and needed to be treated as such. Their message was not clear to me at first, but after several meetings I began to realize that these crazy people did not want anything from me. They really believed the words they read at every meeting—that their main goal was to carry the message to the addict who still suffers. Hey, that was *me*!

There were no dues or fees, no shirts or hats to wear. No background checks, interviews, drug tests, or physical exams were required—just the desire to stop using pills. I had never been involved with any group that had such a simple membership requirement or such a clearly defined purpose. They offered me a different way of life by carrying the message to me, and because the message was not being forced on me, I chose to accept it. I have always struggled with authority figures telling me what I need to do. Church, parents, bosses, spouse, co-workers—*they* were the problem, not *me*!

I do not remember all of the details of my first P.A. meeting. I was still using pills because I believed I was having pain. But I do remember hearing stories at my first P.A. meeting that echoed my exact thoughts about pill using. I heard people say, "I can't tell you how many times I took my last pill," or, "After this prescription I won't need any more," and the one that hit me square between the eyes: "I would replace my spouse's pain pills with regular acetaminophen, so if my spouse looked, the right amount appeared to be in the bottle." I had done exactly that with my wife's pain pills when she went through cancer treatment.

After all of this, though, I still believed I was different from the rest of these pill addicts. I may have had a using *problem*, but they were *addicts*! I was different because I could control my using. I was different because I had what I thought were real pain issues. But I also remember feeling welcome and comfortable around what I felt were "my kind of people," and it seemed as if all they wanted to do was help me, so I stuck around.

I did not come in wanting to work the steps, get a sponsor, or work any other part of the program. I was sure I could do it *my way*. To this day I truly do not remember how many times I relapsed (somewhere between three and five seems right). I know I kept the first couple of relapses secret. When I relapsed, I was abusing my own doctor-prescribed medications and I was once again stealing my wife's pills, which this time had been prescribed after surgery on her broken arm. I remember the shame and utter despair I would feel during these relapses. I wouldn't tell my wife I was stealing her pills until after they were gone. She would be mad but I would be able to get her to come around and forgive me, as she always did. She would be pissed off for a few days, then become concerned for my pain, and then begin to believe me when I said I would control my using from then on.

Finally, when my guilt over these relapses became overwhelming, I had to tell the truth in a meeting. I was not thrown out, scorned, banished, tarred, feathered, or judged. On the contrary, I was completely accepted, and people even thanked me for my honesty. The light started to come on. It was a very freeing experience, relieving me of a tremendous weight. I felt a promise of hope that I had never before experienced. Maybe some of this program actually worked. I now thought I was almost an addict, but still not exactly like the rest of the sorry people in these rooms. After all, I had a job and I was married with kids. I had no legal troubles and no court card that had to be signed. I just knew that with my newfound honesty, I could manage my use of pills, and I was sure I could do that if I kept coming back. I had accepted a part of the P.A. message, but I still had plenty of reservations.

My last relapse happened during a time when everything seemed to be going well. My wife had left for the weekend to visit her mom. I did not need any pain meds as I had fully recovered from surgeries. I was feeling great and getting a lot done. Then, as I walked past the jewelry box where my wife hid her meds, it almost seemed as if the pills were calling to me: "Think about how much we could get done together—and while you're at it, I'll give you a buzz, too." Of course, it was not the pills talking—it was my addict mind. It seemed like a great idea. I would use just four of the thirty or so she had, two today and two tomorrow. "Oh, what a great plan," I thought, "So much will get done, and a buzz to boot." I took two right away to jump-start the production train. I had a little guilt in the back of my mind, but I brushed it aside, thinking of all the good that would come from this great plan! The two pills lasted about forty-five minutes and then the tingly buzz started to fade away. That could affect production, so two more were in order. This cycle continued and very little of the to-do list got done. When the pills were gone, I was dope sick—and sick with guilt.

When I told my wife what I had done, she was furious, but for the first time I did not care what she thought. *I was finally sick and tired of being sick and tired.* I told her she could not be any more disappointed or angry than I was. This fell on deaf ears, as I am sure I had used these lines many times before, but for me it was different. This time I really meant it.

There was a P.A. meeting the next day, which also happened to be my birthday. I was excited, and eager to go and tell on myself. I was finally ready to give up and surrender to the program. My P.A. brothers and sisters, as usual, welcomed me back with love and understanding. When I heard the words, "Each group has but one primary purpose—to carry the message to the addict who still suffers," I had an important realization. The group was actually a power greater than me, and this power was sending me a message. The message hit me in the head like a frying pan. I was no different than anyone else in the room. I had no control over my addiction, and my life was totally unmanageable, but if I believed in these other addicts, and took the Twelve Steps they suggested, I could stop using pills and find a new way of life, just as they were doing. Today, I cling to this group that saved my life, and I am beginning to know the joy that comes from reaching out to newcomers and sharing the message of recovery with addicts who still suffer.

WORKING TRADITION FIVE

The Fifth Tradition is our heart and soul. The more we reflect on it, the more we remember that the main reason for our P.A. group's existence is to carry the message of recovery to the pill addict who still suffers. Many of our groups regularly take a group inventory to evaluate how well we are fulfilling our commitment to our primary purpose. We ask ourselves questions such as these, and, based upon our answers, make the necessary changes.

1. How do my group and I make sure that newcomers are warmly welcomed? How many of us stick our hand out and introduce ourselves, or hug someone who is new?

2. Does our group have a greeter, someone whose job it is to welcome everyone to the meeting, paying special attention to welcome newcomers? Do we have someone who makes sure that newcomers are given meeting schedules, phone numbers, and literature?

3. In what ways can my group and I help newcomers feel like they are a part of the natural camaraderie that takes place at our meetings? Why is it so important to make them feel included?

4. What can I do when I am sharing in meetings that will help me to better connect with the pill addict who still suffers?

5. How often do I go out of my way to talk to someone new instead of just talking to the people I already know? Do we always invite newcomers to join us for coffee after the meeting, or to come along on picnics or other group activities?

6. How and why do we give special treatment to visiting members of our fellowship from other groups in our area, or from out of town?

7. How well do I listen to everyone who shares? How can I be more attentive and more responsive to members who are not new, but are going through a difficult time?

8. How is the atmosphere of recovery in our group right now? How do I contribute to the atmosphere of recovery in my group? Are there changes my group and I can make to improve that atmosphere?

9. How does our group use our public information and hospitals and institutions sub-committees to assist us in reaching more pill addicts who still suffer? What else can we do to inform more suffering pill addicts about our meeting and attract them to attend?

10. In what ways do I let others carry more of the load than is necessary or fair? What can I personally do as a member of my group to further our primary purpose in some of the ways listed above?

TRADITION SIX

"A P.A. group ought never endorse, finance, or lend the P.A. name to any related facility or outside enterprise, lest problems of money, property, or prestige divert us from our primary purpose."

Tradition Six sets some clear boundaries for keeping our groups focused on their primary purpose, which is defined in Tradition Five as carrying the message of recovery to the pill addict who still suffers. Why are these boundaries necessary? As pill addicts, most of us tend to overcomplicate things and blow them out of proportion, even in recovery. It is no accident that two of the slogans we hear most frequently in our program are, "Keep it simple," and "Easy does it." Another common symptom of our disease is our inability to focus—many of us are very easily distracted. Tradition Six cautions our groups about the consequences of getting involved with any endeavor that might dilute the message of Pills Anonymous or detract from its mission.

The restrictions of Tradition Six apply to our groups and to P.A. as a whole, but not to our individual members. As individuals, we are free to give our time and/or money to hospitals, recovery homes, schools, charities, or any other humanitarian endeavors we choose. Individually, we can go to work for a treatment center, start a sober-living home, or set up a recovery-oriented clubhouse. These are all worthy projects, and we are free to pursue them as we wish, but we must always remember that when we participate in such enterprises, we should do so as individuals and not as representatives of Pills Anonymous.

We may well ask, "What is wrong with Pills Anonymous financing a group home, helping to build a hospital, sponsoring a television show about recovery, or supporting a politician who wants to help pill addicts? What is wrong with P.A. directly endorsing something that is obviously good and wholesome?" Tradition Six explains that involving our fellowship with such projects may cause problems—complications that will distract us, draining time and energy away from our main task.

These consequences have been experienced first-hand by other twelve-step groups, and we would be wise to learn from their experiences. This is a spiritual program and we find it hard to be spiritual when we are preoccupied with property, prestige, and money. Pills Anonymous does not require real estate in order to carry its message. It does not hope to be seen as a leader in the field of recovery or become famous for its work with pill addicts. P.A. groups have no need to accumulate money in order to carry the message. Even our "wealthiest" groups that pay rent and provide coffee, refreshments, and literature do not require much in the way of operating funds. According to our traditions, we are fully self-supporting and decline outside contributions, having faith that our Higher Power will supply everything we need to carry out our primary purpose. Our program is simply based on the principle of one pill addict carrying the message to another, and that can take place, if need be, in a public park or private home.

Tradition Six reminds us that Pills Anonymous also has no business approving, or seeking the approval of, related facilities or outside enterprises. We do not try to ride on anyone else's coattails and we do not want anyone riding on ours. We do pay a fair rental amount for our meeting places, but we take care not to endorse or lend our name to that facility. It is not a good idea for our groups' names to include any part of the name of the facility in which we meet because that would be a case of direct affiliation and would constitute an implied endorsement. By the same token, if the facility, whether it is a church, hospital, or recovery home, advertises our meetings in any way, we should try to make them aware that they are compromising the traditions of Pills Anonymous. We cannot demand that they stop using our name because they are not bound by our traditions, but we are obligated to amicably discuss the issue with them, and explain how and why our traditions guide our groups. After this effort, if agreement cannot be reached, the group may decide to move their meeting.

In carrying the message of recovery, our groups will come into contact with people in other organizations, especially those who may work with still-suffering pill addicts. This is healthy. Contact with doctors, clergymen, teachers, friends, relatives, and others can improve public understanding of pill addiction and increase the chances that more pill addicts will hear our message. Our goal is to cooperate, but not affiliate. Let us say for example that a county sheriff invites our group to conduct P.A. meetings in the county jail. This turns out to be a wonderful idea, and many suffering pill addicts are helped through these jailhouse meetings. But then suppose that during the next election, members of our P.A. group want to pass the collection basket at a meeting for donations to the good sheriff's campaign? This might seem like a good idea, but it directly contradicts our Sixth Tradition and compromises our integrity.

Some endorsements can be a bit more complicated. For example, in a meeting schedule or flyer we may want to print the name of the church, hospital, or treatment center in which our meeting takes place so that newcomers can more easily find us. However, this must be weighed against the fact that printing the name of the facility may constitute an implied endorsement by Pills Anonymous. The group might decide that a street address is sufficient to identify the location. On the other hand, the group could conclude that some pill addicts would not find us if we did not mention the facility's name. Another option might be to use the facility's name, but also include a brief statement on the printed piece stating that P.A. is not associated with—and does not endorse—that facility. There is no hard and fast rule on this. According to the Fourth Tradition, our groups are autonomous and must decide these issues for themselves, using the Second Tradition to invoke our only ultimate authority—a loving God as He may express Himself in our group conscience.

Our groups can also avoid creating implied endorsements by making sure that all the literature read during our meetings has been approved by Pills Anonymous. The concept of conference-approved literature was developed by other twelve-step groups, and has been adopted by Pills Anonymous. Literature is reviewed and edited by the P.A. Common Welfare Committee and then submitted to our World Service Conference for approval. Our members are free to read recovery literature from any source, but in keeping with Tradition Six, we should read only Conference-approved literature during our meetings.

Other fellowship literature, such as announcements and newsletters, may be displayed along with Conference-approved literature, but always at the group's discretion. Announcements directly relating to Pills Anonymous are usually read at the end of the meeting, and are clearly labeled as "P.A. announcements." However, if we announce non-P.A. events during a meeting, we are lending the P.A. name to some "related facility or outside enterprise." If we read or display literature created outside the Pills Anonymous

Fellowship, we are contradicting our Sixth Tradition by creating an implied endorsement of some other individual or group. We are sanctioning their primary purpose, not ours. Reading or displaying literature from outside our fellowship may also compromise the clarity of the P.A. message and undermine the principle of unity upon which our personal recovery depends.

The Sixth Tradition also applies to the words we use when we speak during our meetings. For example, if we attend a church or are enrolled in a treatment center, we try not to identify that organization by name when we share so that no implied endorsement occurs. Even though we may attend other twelve-step recovery meetings, when we are at a P.A. meeting, we identify ourselves as pill addicts and talk only about Pills Anonymous when we share, because our goal is to deliver a clear and simple message to the newcomer.

"Live and let live" is another one of our popular slogans. We pill addicts find it difficult to mind our own business. We developed a habit of keeping the focus on others to avoid having to look at ourselves, and we created chaos in all our relationships. We either had to force others to come around to our way of thinking, or we caved-in to their wishes just to please them. Most of us had very little use for principles such as faith, harmony, integrity, humility, and anonymity—character traits that enable us to get along with people instead of alienating them. Yet, it is exactly these principles of selfless service that our groups must regularly practice if we wish to avoid problems with related facilities and outside enterprises that might compromise or even cripple our fellowship. By understanding and applying Tradition Six, we can safeguard the survival of Pills Anonymous—and devote all of our energy to carrying a clear and consistent message of hope to pill addicts seeking recovery.

OUR MEMBERS' EXPERIENCE WITH TRADITION SIX

PROTECTION FROM CONFUSION

Having been in Pills Anonymous for a while, I discovered that many of us have gone through treatment for our addiction to pills and other mind-altering substances, while others have been referred to doctors who deal with addiction to help them get clean. Some of the most amazing recoveries I have watched, and sometimes been a part of, were those of people who got clean by coming to P.A. meetings while slowly tapering off their pills. They may have been sleeping on a friend's couch while trying to raise a child on their own, and had no resources to go to any doctor. Yet with time, they got sponsors and worked the steps, got jobs, served at meetings and beyond, and even went on to hold P.A. World Service Conference positions!

When I came into the rooms, I heard others mention particular doctors who had helped them and others. Personally, I was steered away from medicine as I had gotten almost all of my pills from doctors. My life and addiction were wrapped up in the routine of going to doctors, and sometimes having procedures, all to get more pills. Several years into my recovery, we had people coming into the rooms of P.A. who were still using pills but wanted to get clean. Some of our home group members suggested that we have a list of specialty doctors to hand out to these people. It was brought up at our group business meeting and, because of Tradition Six, we decided not to do this because this list of physicians would be an endorsement of outside enterprises. We also agreed that as individuals, we could privately share the names of specific doctors, treatment centers, or counselors with other addicts on a one-to-one basis, but we should not endorse such outside resources during a meeting or as a group.

Tradition Six protected us as a group, and also protected the newcomer who was still suffering. If we had put that list out, it would have been an endorsement, and others may have wanted to put out treatment center brochures, counseling referrals, lists of psychiatrists, dentists, and so on. The end result would have presented a very confusing and diluted message to the newcomer, and also could have caused problems of money, property, and prestige because of our association with these outside resources. If I had come into a meeting as a newcomer, and had seen a list of doctors recommended by the group, I would have jumped to grab the list and call for an appointment before the doctor's office even opened. I may have gone to each and every doctor on the list to get something to kill the pain of those overwhelming feelings we must endure when we stop taking pills. I do not believe I would have found the strength and hope I needed at the meetings or gotten a sponsor—and I most likely would have relapsed.

Tradition Six shields us as a group and as individuals, keeping us focused on our primary purpose as we grow. Unencumbered, we thrive—and are able to carry the message to the pill addict who still suffers.

WORKING TRADITION SIX

The Sixth Tradition provides our groups with guidelines for dealing with other organizations and outlines the hazards that await us if we compromise those principles. While we are free to act in any way we want as individuals, we surrender some of that freedom when we act as members of a Pills Anonymous group. At that point, we become responsible for understanding the traditions and helping our groups to observe them. By answering the following questions, we can improve our understanding of Tradition Six and help to safeguard our groups against diversions from our primary purpose.

1. How does my group deal with the facility in which it holds its meetings? Are there any things we do that might imply an endorsement of that facility? Has the facility ever done anything to imply that they are associated with Pills Anonymous, and how have we dealt with that?

2. Other than our meeting facility, does my group have contact with other outside organizations or enterprises? Have we ever done anything that might imply we endorse those entities or are associated with them in any way?

3. How well does my group deal with professionals, relatives, or friends who might help us deliver our message of hope to the pill addict who still suffers? Have any issues of money, property, or prestige ever arisen, and how did we apply the Sixth Tradition to those situations? What experiences have I had in applying the Sixth Tradition?

4. How do my group and I relate to other twelve-step groups? In what ways do we cooperate with them? What steps do we take to make sure that our relationship is not seen as an affiliation?

5. How well do I think my group understands the Sixth Tradition? What can I do to help the group expand its understanding?

6. Do I observe the Sixth Tradition when sharing at meetings? In what ways?

7. What does my group do to encourage its members to observe the Sixth Tradition when sharing at meetings? If, for example, someone mentions another organization

or institution by name, do we gently bring the Sixth Tradition to their attention after the meeting?

8. Why is it important to observe the First Tradition (our common welfare coming first) and the Twelfth Tradition (placing principles before personalities) whenever we discuss a possible breach of the Sixth Tradition?

9. How does Tradition Six apply to the literature we make available at our meetings? How well do the members of my group and I understand the concept of Conference-approved literature, and the reasoning behind it?

10. Faith, harmony, integrity, humility, and anonymity are all important spiritual principles that we need to practice in our observance of the Sixth Tradition. How well do my group and I apply each one?

11. In my own daily life, how can I apply these spiritual principles (faith, harmony, integrity, humility, and anonymity) to improve my relationships with others?

TRADITION SEVEN

"Every P.A. group ought to be fully self-supporting, declining outside contributions."

Tradition Six cautions our groups to refrain from funding, endorsing, or lending the Pills Anonymous name to related facilities or outside enterprises so that we are not distracted from our primary purpose. But what if related facilities, outside organizations, or non-P.A. members want to contribute to help support our efforts? This may not seem like such a bad idea, but our Seventh Tradition clearly states that we should be fully self-supporting and refuse all contributions from any outside organizations or individuals.

This is quite a departure for many pill addicts. When we were using pills, we consistently avoided taking full responsibility for our own lives. Under the influence of mind-altering substances, we tended to spend money with reckless abandon. Deluded by our disease, we expected other people and institutions to support us, taking advantage of them whenever we thought we could get away with it. Driven by the self-centeredness of addiction, we often acted like leeches, draining the resources of our families, friends, and communities. When one source brushed us off, we simply moved on to the next victim. Blinded by selfishness, we actually viewed ourselves as the victims, believing that we were fully entitled to everything we could beg, borrow, or steal.

In recovery, we learn the benefits of managing our financial affairs honestly and responsibly, doing the necessary footwork and trusting our Higher Power for the results. Once a burden on society, we are now earning the right to stand on our own, secure in the faith that a power greater than ourselves will always provide whatever we really need. Our Pills Anonymous Fellowship takes exactly the same stance, relying only on its own membership for support.

Tradition Seven advises that our groups decline all outside contributions. This means we accept contributions only from members of Pills Anonymous. It also means that the only requirement for giving financial support to our fellowship is to be a member of P.A. According to our Third Tradition, membership is a matter determined solely by the individual. Those new to P.A. may take some time to decide on their membership, so our groups generally let newcomers know they are under no obligation to contribute when the basket is passed.

For members, it is a different story. While no member should ever be made to feel that contributions are mandatory, many of us see the Seventh Tradition as a way to express our gratitude to the fellowship that literally saved our lives. This program encourages us to become responsible and productive members of society. What better place to begin than in our own meeting rooms? By contributing to our groups, we help sustain and strengthen them, improving their ability to effectively carry the message of recovery to all pill addicts, including ourselves. When we observe the Seventh Tradition, we are also enriching ourselves spiritually by taking on responsibility, expressing our gratitude, and demonstrating faith in a Higher Power. If P.A. accepted outside contributions, we would be deprived of some of the spiritual benefits we experience by supporting our own fellowship.

There are many reasons for not accepting outside donations. Our predecessors in other twelve-step programs learned the hard way that accepting outside contributions can lead to disunity and controversy. Money often comes with strings attached. As an old saying goes, "He who pays the piper calls the tune." All too often, an act of generosity is followed by a suggestion or demand that the money be spent in a certain way. Let us say, for example, that a pharmaceutical company offers P.A. a free publicity campaign, to be focused on The Twenty Questions (P.A.'s list of questions that people can use to determine if they are pill addicts). While working on the campaign the company suggests a slight change in the wording of the questions to improve their presentation of our combined messages. Not wishing to offend our potential benefactors, we might consider making this minor modification, thinking that, after all, the benefits of the publicity campaign far outweigh the consequences of changing a few words of our message. Yet this is the P.A. message that saved our own lives and the lives of many other pill addicts. By tampering with it, we may dilute or change it, and in the end make it less effective. The Seventh Tradition protects us from heading down this slippery slope. If we allow outside individuals or organizations to contribute to Pills Anonymous, we risk incurring obligations and compromising our integrity. We risk the freedom that we have so painstakingly gained.

Simplicity is a quality that can actually improve our ability to carry the message of recovery, so we view having too much money as more of a problem for our groups than having too little. Our groups really do not need very much to function. The Seventh Tradition collection is used to pay for rent and literature first, and if anything is left over, the group may use that money to purchase refreshments and financially support Pills Anonymous service boards and committees.

On occasion, we may not have enough to pay for rent and literature, and members who can afford it will give a little bit extra—but not too much extra. A large donation from one individual can deprive other members of the benefits of sharing responsibility for the group's support. It can also compromise the principle of anonymity by calling special attention to the donor, who the group might then perceive as more important or influential than its other members. An overly generous donor also risks developing an inappropriate sense of his own importance to the group. Anonymity is the spiritual foundation of all our traditions, and when it comes to money, we are wise to avoid any situation that might tempt us to place personalities before principles.

The principles of the Seventh Tradition can be applied to all contributions, not just money. We can also contribute to our fellowship through our personal service — setting up chairs, making coffee, greeting newcomers, sharing at meetings, sponsoring others, participating in business meetings, or serving as secretary, treasurer, or group representative. Just as we encourage our members to take equal responsibility when it comes to giving money, we also try to fairly share these non-monetary contributions. We spread our service positions among as many members as we can, and rotate these positions whenever possible so that no one becomes entrenched in a particular role. When we share at meetings, we try to limit our time so that all others have an equal chance to speak. And just as with money, there is often a fine line between giving too much and too little of our time and energy. As always, we must rely on our Higher Power for guidance.

OUR MEMBERS' EXPERIENCE WITH TRADITION SEVEN

AN INVESTMENT IN MY RECOVERY

Having committed to daily recovery meetings after leaving an inpatient treatment facility, I attended Pills Anonymous and other twelve-step meetings as well. I had not yet found "the truth," so one of the first things my old value system zeroed in on was the passing of the Seventh Tradition basket. I carried a lot of feelings of skepticism and cynicism regarding the collection of money. I had belonged to a religious organization that pressured its congregation for financial support, using guilt and the promise of spiritual benefit. I had written a lot of large checks to the church, often while high on pills, and never felt the kind of spiritual relief I thought I should feel as a result. So the first time I saw the Seventh Tradition basket going around, I thought to myself, "Well, here we go again. I knew there had to be a catch." My newly chosen sponsor helped me find a better perspective when he told me that the recovery tools and guidance are free, and that the money just takes care of the overhead. After that I began to let go of my past emotional bias against the collection of money for a cause. In time, I came to believe that the Seventh Tradition was an investment in my recovery and my future, helping me to let go of the past.

As my recovery has progressed over the years, my sponsor and I have noticed that as part of my quest for inner peace, my old superficial, material values are being replaced by a system of spiritual principles. With this change, I have become more invested in the value of my recovery program and my service to this program. There are many things I do to put my money where my mouth is, and live true to my newfound principles. One very simple example is that I no longer buy coffee at an expensive coffeehouse. I discovered that I don't even particularly like the taste of their coffee. I used to buy it there because my friends did and I wanted to do the popular thing. Instead, I purchase my coffee at a local convenience store or make my own coffee at home. I can then put the difference between the expensive coffee and my more frugal choice into the Seventh Tradition basket. I definitely like to drink coffee, so this really adds up!

When I took advantage of the opportunity to involve myself in service for Pills Anonymous, I learned how important it is that we decline outside contributions. For instance, over

the last several years I have served on a planning and or-
ganizing committee to create a large all-day recovery event.
Our responsibilities include such things as printing flyers,
providing food, finding speakers, making decorations, and
renting equipment for the event. On one occasion, a member
who was a salesman for a rental company offered to get us
the equipment we needed at no cost. The committee declined
this offer because the salesman did not own the rental company, so its assets weren't his to contribute. Sometimes when
needs were brought to the committee, as a business owner,
I offered my personal contacts to provide for discounted or
free services to meet those needs. Every time I made such
an offer, one of the old-timers on the committee would say,
"Only if that person is in the program." After a while my ego,
feeling restless and discontented, prompted me to ask what
the big deal was. In answering my question, someone suggested that I re-read the Seventh Tradition, which reminds
us that unless we are providing something through our own
contributions, the result will never be unconditional. Our
event has always been successful, both financially and as a
way to carry the message of recovery, and we've done just
fine declining outside contributions. Like my sponsor always
says of the event, "Breaking even is the hard part. After that,
it is all gravy."

Through this and other experiences, I have learned that
practicing the Seventh Tradition helps me to be responsible
for taking care of myself—probably for the first time in my
life. My primary purpose in recovery is to find peace of mind.
Outside contributions or influences usually have strings attached in the real world. Those strings could be pulled by a
person or organization whose primary purpose might differ
from ours, causing problems of control that result in confusion, negativity, and needless drama. I created enough of
that myself in the past, and I don't need any of that in my
recovery today.

WORKING TRADITION SEVEN

In general, our fellowship tends to minimize the importance of money, preferring to focus on the spiritual enrichment we find in the Twelve Steps. Fortunately the Seventh Tradition stands as a spiritual beacon, helping us to chart a safe course when navigating our way through financial waters. When our groups are fully self-supporting, they remain autonomous and free, beholden to no one, except a loving God as He may express Himself in our group conscience. The following questions may help us examine how well we, as individual members, and our group are following the principles of the Seventh Tradition.

1. What would happen if my group could not pay its rent? What actions have we taken to ensure that we are able to meet our financial obligations (like establishing a prudent reserve)?

2. Does my group let newcomers know that they are not obligated to contribute when the basket is passed? Why is it important to share this information with newcomers?

3. If any members have made disproportionately large contributions, how did my group deal with the situation?

4. How should the members of my group and I respond when non-members wish to make a donation? What are some of the possible consequences of accepting donations from non-members? What can we do to educate non-members about our Seventh Tradition?

5. How does my group prioritize its expenditures at our business meetings?

6. How do we make our members aware that our service boards need financial support to properly carry out the work our groups have delegated to them?

7. How and why does the practice of rotating service positions reflect the Seventh Tradition? What spiritual principles are applied in this process?

8. How many service positions does my group have, and how often do we rotate them? Should we rotate any of these positions more or less frequently? How can we get more members involved so that they too will experience the rewards of selfless service? How do I apply this concept in my own service?

9. In what ways do I support my group? What more can I do to support our groups, service bodies, or the P.A. Fellowship as a whole?

10. Do I view my contributions—monetary and other-wise—as an opportunity or an obligation? How does being financially responsible enrich my recovery?

11. How can I apply the spiritual principles of the Seventh Tradition (faith, responsibility, integrity, simplicity, generosity, and anonymity) to improve my own handling of money?

TRADITION EIGHT

"Pills Anonymous should remain forever nonprofessional, but our service centers may employ special workers."

Pills Anonymous is a nonprofit fellowship of men and women who meet regularly to share their experience, strength, and hope. Through these efforts, we help each other remain free from pill addiction, and we carry the message of recovery to pill addicts who still suffer. This is who we are, and this is all we are.

Tradition Eight says unequivocally that we are not professionals when we are acting on behalf of Pills Anonymous. When sharing at a meeting, speaking about P.A. at a local hospital, or sponsoring another member, we are always nonprofessionals. We refrain from claiming that we are trained experts in recovery, and we neither seek nor accept payment for our efforts. Of course, in their personal pursuits, many of our members accumulate professional credentials and earn commensurate salaries as doctors, lawyers, teachers, counselors, clergymen, and so forth; but when it comes to P.A., our vocations are completely irrelevant. As members of P.A., our only qualification is our own personal experience with recovery from pill addiction, and our only compensation should be the spiritual satisfaction we gain from carrying the message of recovery to others.

A person may be called a professional when he is highly skilled at what he does. In Pills Anonymous, no one is identified as an expert in recovery, and nobody earns a degree or certificate for not using pills. We may receive some recognition from our group in the form of a "chip" or key tag, and perhaps a slice of cake when we celebrate our clean date, but the real purpose of this celebration is to share hope with newcomers. "The world record for staying clean is twenty-four hours, because we only stay clean one day at a time." This saying reminds us to remain humble and to never take our recovery for granted. We practice humility by not pretending to have all the answers no matter how much time we have in recovery. As P.A. members, we reject prestige and status, instead embracing the spirit of anonymity, which is the spiritual foundation of our traditions. No member of our fellowship is more important than any other member.

A person may also be called a professional when he gets paid for what he does. In Traditions Six and Seven, we learned that disregarding our traditions can lead to money problems that might interfere with our primary purpose. Tradition Eight also helps guard the purity and effectiveness of our Twelfth Step work (carrying the message to other pill addicts) by completely removing money from the equation. We do Twelfth Step work—such as sponsoring fellow pill addicts, speaking at meetings, or participating in community outreach programs—without being paid for our efforts. This helps ensure that all basic aspects of our recovery remain free. We may at times pay for the transportation or lodging of a member who is engaged in service work, but we do not pay anyone for sharing their experience. If we did this, we would risk transforming a speaker's heartfelt message into a paid performance, thereby turning what should be a labor of love into a quest for profit.

As individuals, we neither want nor need professional certification for the purpose of carrying the message of recovery, and as we learn from the Sixth Tradition, neither do our groups. Our message is completely sufficient in and of itself, without any type of endorsement from any outside entity. We are not affiliated with any hospitals, churches, treatment centers, or clinics. Our groups do not provide medical, legal, psychiatric, or any other professional services. The Pills Anonymous program is simply based on the therapeutic value of one pill addict helping another, so our groups already have just about everything they need to fulfill their primary purpose.

There are, however, occasions when we may need the help of a professional. For example, a committee may require the services of a lawyer, accountant, or graphic artist. There is nothing wrong with paying such an expert, who may or may not be a P.A. member, to assist us in our work. These paid professionals are not P.A. employees. They are not directly responsible to the P.A. Fellowship, and they are not required to follow the Twelve Traditions. Although their work may wind up helping pill addicts who still suffer, the primary purpose of paid professionals is to do a good job for their clients and, in the process, earn money for themselves and their companies.

The Eighth Tradition does provide for a type of employee that we call a "special worker." These are individuals who may or may not be members of P.A., and are hired by what we refer to as a "service center." Our traditions provide for the creation of, "service boards or committees directly responsible to those they serve," and a service center is simply a place where the work of such service boards or committees takes place. These service centers are meant to perform functions that our service boards, committees, and groups may not be equipped to handle. These tasks might include maintaining fellowship-wide communication, publishing and distributing books and literature, responding to inquiries from the general public, and putting on special events.

Clubhouses, recovery homes, or halfway houses are not considered service centers since they are not part of the Pills Anonymous service structure, and their employees are not considered P.A. special workers. In this electronic age, many services may not even require brick-and-mortar facilities, so our definition of service centers may be expanded to include the performance of functions that do not require a physical space.

We try to staff our service centers, boards, or committees with unpaid volunteers, but volunteers can only do so much. For this reason we may need to employ special workers to assist us. Special workers may include receptionists, secretaries, office managers, or warehouse workers. They may also be certified professionals such as accountants or lawyers, or provide professional management or communications services. Regardless of the work they do, when they are paid employees of Pills Anonymous, their status changes to that of special workers. As such, they are required to do their work in accordance with the Twelve Traditions and are accountable to the service board or committee for which they work. As a result, they are indirectly responsible to the Pills Anonymous Fellowship as a whole. Special workers may or may not be P.A. members, depending on the nature of the job they are performing. Although we may sincerely wish to help recovering pill addicts by giving them jobs, when it comes to hiring and compensating special workers, our primary consideration must be their ability to perform their duties. In addition, special workers who are P.A. members should not be paid any less than non-members because of the misguided belief that, "they should be glad to be of service."

Tradition Eight effectively separates Twelfth Step work from paid jobs in Pills Anonymous. Because of this distinction, we are able to keep our motives pure when we do service work. When there is no financial compensation involved, it is far easier for us to be truly selfless, and to enjoy the unparalleled spiritual rewards of freely reaching out to help other pill addicts.

OUR MEMBER'S EXPERIENCE WITH TRADITION EIGHT

BEING A DOCTOR DOESN'T DEFINE ME

I'm a hard-core pill addict. I took lots of pills and they almost killed me. I also happen to be a medical professional—specifically, a doctor. These particular credentials did not help me get into recovery any faster than if I had been involved in any other occupation. In fact, I would say being a doctor may have been my downfall because I thought I was so smart that I could figure out "this little pill problem" on my own. With the rigorous training I received as a child to be totally self-sufficient, and with an endless supply of will-power, it didn't cross my mind that asking for help might be something to consider.

By God's grace I ended up in an inpatient rehabilitation facility, and then found the rooms of Pills Anonymous. This was certainly not my plan, but as I have come to realize, my Higher Power usually does for me what I can't or won't do for myself! When I first came into the rooms, I wasn't quite convinced I needed you "crazy people" to help me stay clean. I didn't initially share about being a doctor—not out of humility or respect, but because I just didn't want you to think less of me or my profession. And I definitely didn't want you crazy people to pity me!

I did know that I didn't want to use again. I didn't want to be the suicidal, lonely, soulless being I had become by using pills. So I did what you said, got a sponsor, and worked the steps. I was quite astonished that my first sponsor was not at all impressed by or in awe of working with someone of my background and credentials. At times I felt she treated me like a child. Now I realize that she treated me like a child because I was acting like one!

I didn't know much about the traditions until after I had worked the steps, so I wasn't aware of the principles underlying the Eighth Tradition until a few years into my recovery. However, I did become acutely aware of one aspect of this tradition early in my recovery when another member found out I was a doctor and asked me to call in a prescription for his pill of choice right after a P.A. meeting! I experienced intense feelings of anxiety from this encounter. After all, I wrote prescriptions for that particular medication many times during the course of a normal workday. I realized that the person who asked me for the prescription must have been in a great deal of mental anguish to have the nerve to ask for such a thing, especially after a P.A. meeting. I quickly talked to some other members and called my sponsor, as I was taught to do. Although I didn't realize it at the time, my sponsor and those other members taught me a little bit about the Eighth Tradition that night. My sponsor reminded me that when I'm at a twelve-step meeting, I'm first and foremost a recovering addict. I'm not a doctor or therapist and I'm not a drug dealer. I'm there to listen to and share my experience, strength, and hope, not my DEA number.

A few years into recovery, I had another experience which relates to the Eighth Tradition. It is not unusual for students (and sometimes practitioners) in medical, psychological, or social services programs to visit a meeting to learn more about the twelve-step process. On one occasion a practicing counselor visited our meeting. He was very gracious, refrained from sharing, and seemed to have some knowledge about the workings of twelve-step groups. However, after the meeting he promptly started handing out his card, looking for prospective clients! Thanks to Tradition Eight, we were able to very kindly stop him in his tracks and explain why this was breaking some very important traditions of our program. Of course, if it had been up to me, I may not have been as gracious as some of the other P.A. members. My Higher Power tends to look out for me at those times!

People in recovery sometimes ask me about specific medical issues. If it's about addiction, I usually remind them that I'm not an addiction specialist, but that I would be happy to talk to them about Pills Anonymous, the steps, and my experiences in recovery. If they approach me about other medical issues, I might offer some very basic information and encourage them to see their medical professional. I have come to realize that my profession is obviously part of my life and my story, but it doesn't have to be included every time I share my experience, strength, and hope. I've also learned that being a doctor doesn't define me—it's my job.

I pray every day for love, tolerance, and compassion, so I can do my work as a doctor according to God's will—and so that I may help the addict who still suffers. I pray to be available to help my family and friends, my coworkers, and any other spiritual beings I meet in the course of this human experience. I don't have to be a doctor to be helpful to others. I do have to live in God's will and keep working on my recovery and spirituality. I always remind myself that the traditions help us to stay focused on our main purpose, which is to help other pill addicts. If nothing else, the traditions remind me of the spiritual principles of this program. They remind me to strive for humility, and to be of service. And God knows I need all the reminders I can get!

WORKING TRADITION EIGHT

Tradition Eight may seem complicated and difficult to understand, especially when we are new in the program or do not have much experience with service work. Answering these questions and dis-cussing them with our sponsor may help to clarify this tradition, and help us understand the importance of separating Twelfth Step work from paid service in P.A.

1. How would my recovery be different if I had been required to pay others for sharing their recovery experience, strength, and hope? How would I view my sponsor if I was charged by the hour for his or her time?

2. Do I sometimes try to sound like an expert on pill addiction and, if so, in what ways? In what ways do I exaggerate my understanding of recovery, when I talk with people both inside and outside our fellowship?

3. On what occasions have I pretended to be an expert on other things, such as medicine, psychiatry, sociology, finance, or spiritual matters?

4. How has my tendency to be a know-it-all affected my relationships with others, both in the program and in other relationships and situations?

5. How have I used the spiritual principles of humility, anonymity, and integrity to counteract my tendency to be arrogant?

6. Have I been involved in service with a group or committee that was reluctant to seek professional advice? How did we—or I—help to apply the Eighth Tradition?

7. In what ways am I personally still reluctant to seek medical, legal, or other kinds of professional help even though it might be a good idea? How might this relate to the way I treated professionals, especially medical professionals, in my pill addiction?

8. What are some of the differences between contracted or consulting professionals and special workers employed by P.A.?

9. Why is it important for our service boards or committees to exercise the spiritual principle of prudence when hiring professionals or special workers?

10. Why is it important that our special workers be paid "the going rate" for their work, even though they may be P.A. members?

11. How often does it cross my mind that I should receive some recognition or reward (even if it is not money) for my efforts to carry the message? How can I become free of these self-serving thoughts?

12. How do I show my gratitude for having received the gift of recovery completely free of charge?

TRADITION NINE

"P.A., as such, ought never be organized, but we may create service boards or committees directly responsible to those they serve."

Most organizations, like governments, corporations, or churches, have rules and a top-down command structure that regulates the activities of its members. Pills Anonymous is different. Our members are free to think, speak, and act as they please. The Twelve Steps are presented as suggestions, and if we do not follow them, our fellow P.A. members do not penalize us—in fact, they welcome us even more warmly, and encourage us to "keep coming back." The consequences of returning to active pill addiction are more motivation for our members than any punishment our fellowship could ever impose.

The Twelve Traditions that guide our groups are also suggestions. P.A. has no enforcement mechanism to ensure that members and groups follow our traditions. Our experience has shown us that when we act without regard for the traditions, we risk disunity and the possible destruction of the fellowship upon which our personal recovery depends. Safeguarding our fellowship is paramount, but our Second Tradition advises us not to rely on any kind of governing body for protection. Instead, it suggests we place our trust in a loving God as He may express Himself in our group conscience, and to rely on our leaders to serve our fellowship rather than govern it.

Our Ninth Tradition clearly states that Pills Anonymous should never be organized, but also recognizes that some sort of structure is necessary to carry the message to as many pill addicts as possible. The most important and effective way we carry our message is in our meetings, by one pill addict sharing with another. This is what we mean by "P.A., as such." Yet there are many other ways to help carry the message, ways that our individual groups would find difficult, burdensome, or impractical. For example, we may wish to maintain phone line programs, conduct panels at hospitals and institutions, provide a single point of contact for the public, or publish books, literature, and meeting directories. We need some way for our groups to carry out these secondary services, leaving them free to focus on their own core mission.

But what kind of service structure would work for recovering pill addicts? Putting one pill addict in charge of another seems like a sure-fire way to harm both. In our disease, we habitually sought control, selfishly manipulating people and situations. We were resentful of any person or organization that had the audacity to try to regulate us. Some of us recklessly defied authority at every step. Our arrogance separated us from family, friends, and society; all our relationships were filled with chaos and conflict. How can we expect such chronically dysfunctional people to band together and form an organization to effectively help others?

The Ninth Tradition gives us a way to achieve this seemingly impossible task, providing for the creation of "service boards or committees directly responsible to those they serve." Through this system, groups can delegate these additional services when they see a clear need, and when they are unable to efficiently perform these services themselves. The Ninth Tradition defines our service structure. Our most basic unit is still the individual member, and members come together to form groups. As a group grows in size, some of its members may create new groups, and as these new groups grow, they may in turn expand into more groups. To maintain unity within the fellowship, a number of groups in the same geographical area may elect members to form a committee or service board that meets periodically to coordinate services, share information, and help one another to find solutions for problems that arise in the individual groups.

As newcomers, we learned that when two or more recovering pill addicts get together, they become much stronger than they were as disconnected individuals. Similarly, when our groups pool their resources to form service boards and committees, they can accomplish a lot more together than they can individually. Groups assign tasks to our service bodies through elected representatives, and the activities of our service boards and committees are reported back to the groups through these same trusted servants. Area service boards and committees may in turn create regional service entities as necessary, which may then form a world service organization to hold world conventions, publish P.A. literature, and carry out similar tasks that cannot be efficiently handled by area or regional service bodies.

It is important to note that Tradition Nine separates Pills Anonymous "as such" from its service boards and committees. "P.A. as such," is simply groups of pill addicts holding meetings to carry the message of recovery. No more, no less. The Fourth Tradition suggests that these P.A. groups should never be organized, remaining completely free to act on their own individual group conscience, except in matters affecting other groups or the fellowship as a whole. Service boards and committees may be created at the discretion of these independent groups of pill addicts, but the service system should not be confused with Pills Anonymous "as such." This is an important distinction. The Pills Anonymous Fellowship may exist without any service structure at all, but service bodies cannot be created or continue to function without Pills Anonymous.

Having our service structure operate apart from our P.A. groups is vital to our spiritual growth. If we blur the line between the two, disputes and controversies that arise in service work may find their way into our meetings and distract us from carrying a clear message of hope and recovery to the pill addict who still suffers. For this reason, our groups have generally found it appropriate to hold their business meetings (during which service issues are discussed) at a separate time from their regular meetings.

Our Ninth Tradition authorizes us to create a service system, but we must remember to apply the spiritual principles we have learned in recovery when we are involved in service work. Simplicity, for example, is essential. Creating an unnecessarily elaborate array of committees and subcommittees might wind up entangling us in a web of bureaucracy, diverting us from our primary purpose. We must also remain prudent, avoiding the temptations of ambition. We should take care not to overreach ourselves, lest we foolishly waste our limited resources. We do not need to expand just to become bigger—but we do seek to grow if it will help us to more widely and effectively fulfill our primary purpose. Diligence is another principle we must exercise to ensure that continual communication is maintained between our groups and the service boards and committees they create.

The spiritual principle of anonymity encourages us to share and rotate our service positions amongst ourselves so that the trappings of pride do not dilute the purity of our selfless service. Perhaps the most useful principle we can remember in our service work is humility, for without it we would be unable to "live and let live," and get along with our fellow trusted servants. Humility is also essential for maintaining harmonious relationships between our service bodies and the entities that created them. We must always remember that Pills Anonymous does not exist to cater to its service boards and committees. On the contrary, our service boards and committees exist solely to serve Pills Anonymous, allowing us to help save the lives of pill addicts by sharing our message of recovery.

Our Members' Experience with Tradition Nine

I Never Did Take Direction Very Well

As a newcomer, I was very suspicious of anyone who wanted to help me, and of the fellowship in general. What kind of weird outfit had I joined? I could see that it was organized, but not like any other organization I had ever known. There appeared to be no rules, only suggestions. If you screwed up, nobody got on your case. Instead, they gave you a hug and told you to keep coming back. Everything seemed upside-down compared to other organizations. For example, I was told that newcomers are the most important people at meetings. Since I was a newcomer, I liked that a lot. I was also told that no one person was really in charge. They said that the people elected to various positions in the fellowship are called "trusted servants," and that these leaders aren't supposed to tell anyone what to do or how to do it. That suited me just fine. I never did take direction very well.

I spent my whole life rebelling against authority. I always felt like I was different from everyone else. When I was four years old, my family moved from the country where I was born to another country, where I felt like a fish out of water. My parents divorced a couple of years later and I stayed with my dad, who remarried and moved the family once again. I continued to feel like I did not fit in, both at school and at home. Dad was a doctor and worked long hours, spending little time with me. My young stepmother gave most of her attention and affection to the two daughters she had with my father. Fearful and mistrustful of both my teachers and peers, I was always getting into trouble at school. Although I got good grades for my studies, I got bad grades for my behavior—for breaking the rules and for not "working and playing well with others."

I went off to college and, free from parental authority for the first time, started binge-drinking on the weekends, lasting only about four months before dropping out. Then the 1960s happened. Suddenly, being different and rebellious was cool. I joined the hippies and started taking and selling drugs of every kind. I loved the way these mind-altering chemicals made me feel, and I loved the newfound respect my peers (especially the opposite sex) began to show me. It got out of hand pretty quickly though, and I was soon injecting drugs of all kinds. I "visited" jails and mental institutions, and came pretty close to dying a couple of times. Angry with the world, myself, my dad, and the women who would not stay with me, I tried to commit suicide three times. After my last unsuccessful attempt, I found religion and got married, but soon became addicted again, this time to prescription pills.

Although I had become a "functional" addict, my life was increasingly chaotic. My deep-seated resentment of any form of authority got me in a lot of hot water with my bosses, the government, and law enforcement. My inability to get along with other people left me with few friends and a failing marriage. By the time I finally became desperate enough to attend my first twelve-step meeting, my life was a shambles. My wife had left me and I was in poor health because of my drug use. I also owed a considerable amount of money in back taxes and had outstanding warrants. Little did I know that I would have to accept an entirely new way of life in order to remain free from active pill addiction, but I was willing to do just about anything to escape from my despondency. My sponsor suggested that I do service work (whatever that was), so I did.

During my early years in service, I made many mistakes. The first time I was elected as the secretary of a meeting, I fancied that I was in charge and could make decisions without consulting the group. I asked some youngsters from a group home to leave because our meeting was supposed to be open only to addicts. My sponsor and other members of the group had to explain the Third Tradition to me, which says that our only requirement for membership is a desire to stop using, something which can only be determined by the individual and no one else.

My arrogance also surfaced when I joined various committees. I was impatient with the slow, seemingly inefficient process the committee used to make its decisions, which then always had to be taken back to the groups to make sure their wishes were being followed. When I voiced my opinion, other members reminded me of the Ninth Tradition, which emphasizes that our service boards and committees are directly responsible to those they serve. After staying in one service position for several years because "nobody else could do it as well as me," I had to swallow my pride and turn over my position to another member of the fellowship. When I complained to my sponsor, he suggested I read Tradition Nine again, which reminds us that this is not a traditional organization. This is not a place where I can feed my sense of self-importance by trying to become indispensable. In doing service work, I have to try to leave my ego behind and recognize that it is a privilege to serve my fellow members, a privilege that I should gladly share.

Gradually, over time, as I worked the Twelve Steps and remained in service, I got a better understanding of the Twelve Traditions. I especially appreciate Tradition Nine, which is so important in keeping our fellowship free from the politics and power struggles that are common in so many other organizations. I am extremely grateful for Tradition Nine because it helps us to focus on carrying P.A.'s simple message of hope to the suffering pill addict—the very same message that I responded to when I was a newcomer.

WORKING TRADITION NINE

Our service structure, as defined by the Ninth Tradition, allows Pills Anonymous to extend its message beyond our group meetings to pill addicts who might otherwise die. If we want to participate in this very rewarding service work, we will want to familiarize ourselves with Tradition Nine and its implications. Answering these questions may deepen our understanding of service work in general, and may also clarify our own roles in helping to carry the message outside the rooms of Pills Anonymous.

1. In what ways am I wary of the organizational aspect of Pills Anonymous? What are some of the problems that have arisen in the service boards and committees I have been a part of, and how were they dealt with? What was my role in those situations and how did they affect my own recovery?

2. How have my past resentments against authority and organizations affected my service work? Do I still sometimes become resentful when my ideas are not accepted? Do I consider other members' suggestions with sufficient respect?

3. What are some occasions on which I have had to exercise humility and patience in service work?

4. In what instances have I been arrogant in my dealings with other members of the fellowship while engaged in service work?

5. How much do I still crave praise for my service work, or have I learned to be of service without such expectations?

6. How gracefully have I given up the service positions I have held, especially the ones I enjoyed the most?

7. When and how do I begin to look for and train a possible replacement to fill a service position I hold? Have there been occasions when I have had to step down from a service position and found that my replacement was not prepared to take on that position? What are some of the steps I can take to help prevent that situation from recurring?

8. Is my group aware of the importance of replacing someone who has held a service position for more than one term—or even for several terms? What are some of the consequences of not observing the principle of service rotation, and how does this relate to the spiritual principle of anonymity?

9. How well does my group maintain ties with other groups in our area, sharing ideas and helping each other when necessary?

10. In business meetings, how often does my group talk about the efforts of our area, regional, and world service boards and committees? How often do we talk about things we can do outside our meetings to carry the message of Pills Anonymous?

TRADITION TEN

"Pills Anonymous has no opinion on outside issues; hence the P.A. name ought never be drawn into public controversy."

In this world, controversy and conflict are inevitable. Throughout history, when disagreements have arisen between individuals, tribes, nations, races, and other groups, fighting has often ensued. Sometimes the conflict is just verbal, and at other times it results in physical confrontation that can lead to destruction and death. The purpose of the Tenth Tradition is to help our groups—and Pills Anonymous as a whole—to avoid the disruptive consequences of conflict. This tradition helps us steer clear of situations and issues that do not directly pertain to our own program. We believe this helps prevent our fellowship from being drawn into any outside debates that might damage our reputation or distract us from our primary purpose of helping pill addicts who still suffer.

As individuals, we are naturally competitive and opinionated. We take sides on political, social, and religious issues, root for our favorite teams, and have different tastes in music and movies. There is, of course, nothing wrong with expressing our individual viewpoints or taking sides—as long as we do not try to force our preferences on others. As individuals, we do not back away from becoming responsible members of society, and we do not refrain from supporting causes we believe to be right. Pills Anonymous, in the spirit of diversity, actually encourages us to stand separately as strong-minded individuals, capable of forming our own opinions and making our own decisions.

Our groups—and Pills Anonymous as a whole—must do just the opposite. By not forming or expressing opinions on outside issues, our fellowship is free to focus sharply on the one thing our members all have in common—the disease of pill addiction and what we can do about it. This stance also nurtures the all-important principle of unity. According to our First Tradition, our common welfare should come first, and our individual recovery depends on P.A. unity. The minute our fellowship decides to take a stand on any outside issue, we endanger that unity, and therefore our individual recovery.

In some ways the Tenth Tradition is like the Tenth Step, which encourages us to continue taking stock of ourselves. Many of us have found that as long as we are busy practicing Step Ten by taking personal inventory, we are far less inclined to take the inventory of others. By focusing on keeping our own side of the street clean, we effectively free ourselves from the cycle of fear, attempted control, frustration, and resentment—a cycle that plagued us in our pill addiction and may continue to trouble us in recovery. Similarly, Tradition Ten implies that P.A. groups should stick to examining their own motivations and actions, not those of other groups or individuals. By tending to our own business, P.A. groups and their service boards and committees become more effective vehicles for carrying out the will of a loving God as expressed in our group conscience.

At times it may be hard to tell the difference between outside issues and legitimate internal concerns. For example, should P.A. have an opinion on the conduct of the pharmaceutical industry or the pill-addiction treatment industry?

Should our trusted servants speak out on behalf of P.A. about the prescription practices of physicians, or on national and state laws? These important issues may be of great concern to individual members of our fellowship, but we must ask ourselves whether they directly affect our groups or P.A. as a whole. We must then ask whether P.A. might be drawn into public controversy by taking a stand or choosing a side on these issues. By expressing an opinion, we risk becoming embroiled in an ongoing conflict, and possibly generating unfavorable publicity. By accepting the guidance of Tradition Ten, we protect P.A. from becoming unnecessarily involved in anything that might tarnish our fellowship's good name and sap our ability to carry out its core mission.

This is not to say that Pills Anonymous will never be drawn into public controversy. We cannot and should not avoid contact with the world around us. Our groups must interact with their meeting facilities, and our service boards and committees will inevitably connect with health professionals, government agencies, and the media. Not everyone will agree with our program, or with all of our ideas. Many outside our fellowship do not accept our proposition that pill addiction is a disease. Others do not share our conviction that we must abstain from all mind-altering substances in order to recover. And what of those who disapprove of the idea that each of us is free to choose a Higher Power of our own understanding? These are clearly "inside" issues, and we should firmly stick to our beliefs on these subjects regardless of any possible public controversy. We cannot deny or compromise the principles and beliefs of our program just because someone disagrees with them.

When confronted we do not back off—but instead, we try to explain our position in a way that does not deliberately incite controversy. In our pill addiction, most of us did not know how to handle conflict. We developed resentments when people contradicted us, or when things did not go our way, or when we did not get something we thought we deserved. Sometimes because of our oversensitive egos, we lashed out with rage at those who got in our way. At other times we avoided confrontation and turned our anger inward, becoming depressed and bitter. Now, in recovery, we must learn how to "disagree without being disagreeable," for our own sake and for the sake of our fellowship.

When we explain the principles of our program, we make it clear that this is what works for us. We avoid trying to convert people to our way of thinking, ever mindful that our public relations policy is based on attraction rather than promotion. We are humble enough to admit that we do not have the answers to all problems. We do not even claim to have the only answer to pill addiction. We try to be cautious when we represent P.A., being careful to be guided by our principles and traditions when informing people about our program. In general, we try to keep a low profile and attempt to avoid any unfavorable coverage by the media. Our ability to help the pill addict who still suffers will be diminished if those still in need are "turned off" to our program because of adverse publicity.

Tradition Ten is intended to guide us in our contacts with the outside world and does not directly apply to what we may or may not say in our recovery gatherings. In our own meeting rooms, we are free to discuss legal, political, social, or moral issues—as long as they pertain directly to our personal recovery. However, we should always be careful about what we say and how we say it. Expressing controversial personal opinions can distract our meetings from their primary purpose. Sharing responsibly means humbly speaking from our own experience, not arrogantly expounding our opinions from the proverbial "soapbox." It means staying in the solution rather than dwelling on the problem, and acknowledging that others may not share our point of view. If we say something potentially divisive in a meeting, we make it clear that we are speaking only for ourselves and not for anyone else in the room or for P.A. as a whole.

It is unrealistic to expect Pills Anonymous or its meetings to always be free of controversy, but by remembering Tradition Ten, we can protect our fellowship from being sidetracked by involvement with irrelevant, non-recovery issues. We can also employ the underlying spiritual principles of this tradition to lessen the impact of any conflict—by speaking and acting prudently and responsibly, being honest about our motivation, and above all, by displaying an attitude of humility and tolerance. When conflicts arise, as they inevitably do, we rely on some of our other traditions to smooth the way for our groups and for the fellowship as a whole. We review Tradition One to make sure we are placing our unity and common welfare first, and we consult Tradition Two to remind ourselves to act in accordance with the wishes of our Higher Power. We consider Tradition Five to determine whether our course of action is satisfying our primary purpose of helping the pill addict who still suffers, and finally, we recall the importance of anonymity, the spiritual principle that always reminds us to place principles before personalities.

OUR MEMBERS' EXPERIENCE WITH TRADITION TEN

RESTRAINT OF TONGUE AND PEN

When I first entered the rooms of Pills Anonymous, I had heard of other twelve-step programs before, but I was not really aware of how they worked, or the principles they encouraged. The first time I saw the Twelve Steps I thought, "Well, great. Now I have to join a 'cult' just to stop using these pills?" Luckily, by no power of my own, I had the open-mindedness to stay, just to check things out. In truth, it all came down to my self-centered desire to not feel as lonely, sad, desperate, and angry as I had for the past few years of my life. I got a sponsor, worked the steps, and—lo and behold—I felt better!

Then I went to a steps and traditions meeting. What's this? Traditions? And there are twelve of them? Am I not busy enough with the steps and service work, not to mention the other aspects of my life like my job and my family?

As has often been the case in my recovery, God gently urged me to take a closer look at the traditions. And by "gently urged me," I mean my sponsor told me to do it. So, I began reading about the traditions. I learned by doing this that being in recovery is not only the greatest blessing I have ever received, but also comes with a great responsibility, which is to be an active member of Pills Anonymous.

This brings me to Tradition Ten. I was like many addicts—not just self-centered and strong-willed, but also extremely nosy, pushy, and opinionated. I thought, "Who cares about being controversial? This is serious business and I don't care what anybody thinks!" Luckily something (God, my sponsor, or probably both!) reminded me of the first nine traditions, particularly Traditions One and Five. Can I help maintain P.A. unity if I am causing controversy that may sully the P.A. name? And how can I possibly carry the message to the newcomer if we have no newcomers because our fellowship has a bad reputation?

I have been blessed with service work that included going to Pills Anonymous and other recovery-based conferences. I have worked at information booths for Pills Anonymous and I have been asked about the fellowship's position on various issues ranging from using antidepressants, to the long-term use of certain opiates for withdrawal, to our stand on legislation regarding DEA restrictions for writing prescriptions for certain narcotics. I have my own opinions about these issues, and very strong opinions about certain issues. But is it my place to discuss my personal opinions regarding these issues when I'm representing Pills Anonymous? Luckily, the Tenth Tradition tells me, "No!"

As I have said, I'm a self-centered, pushy, opinionated addict at my core. Through working the steps and traditions, I am working on these character defects daily and I hope to continue striving to be the kind of person God would have me be rather than what I tend to be. For now, I have to remember that I am human. I may feel very strongly about some things, but when it comes to P.A., I need to remember that this program saved my life, and for that I am extremely grateful. I can express my gratitude by taking some responsibility and trying to help the continued growth of P.A. as a whole. I have made the mistake of trying to force my not-so-humble opinion on other members of P.A. and have seen just how damaging the controversy could be. P.A. does strongly advocate several principles, and it is my responsibility to explain these principles without creating strife. My sponsor always says that if we come from a place of love and tolerance then nothing we say can be wrong. I also have to remember the phrase "restraint of tongue and pen." I have learned that if I pray for God's guidance, I more often say the reasonable, responsible thing. This is especially important to me when representing Pills Anonymous. I try to do my part by being a responsible member of this fellowship because it saved my life—and my greatest hope is that it will save many more lives.

WORKING TRADITION TEN

Simply put, Tradition Ten "keeps our fellowship's nose clean" by keeping it out of other people's business. As individuals, we may form and express opinions on political, legal, social, or moral issues that concern us, but our groups and Pills Anonymous as a whole need to avoid taking stands on these outside issues if we are to remain strongly focused on our primary purpose. Answering these questions may help us to distinguish between "outside" and "inside" issues, and perhaps help us learn the art of saying what we mean without being mean when we say it.

1. What are some examples of "outside" and "inside" issues for Pills Anonymous? How do we tell the difference?

2. What are some of my personal experiences with a group (inside or outside P.A.) that became involved with an irrelevant issue that slowed or halted an important project?

3. Why is it so important that P.A. steer clear of negative publicity? How conscious am I of maintaining a low profile when representing Pills Anonymous, even when I am just paying the rent for our meeting space or standing outside with my fellow members after a meeting?

4. How do I respond when people in the fellowship seek outside help? How can I practice the principles of the Tenth Tradition when I encounter such situations?

5. How do the Sixth, Seventh, and Tenth Traditions protect us from those who might use our meetings to recruit support for their personal causes, or solicit us to purchase an outside product or service? Has this ever happened at a meeting I attended, and how was it handled?

6. What might happen to Pills Anonymous if it strayed from the Tenth Tradition and began taking stances on legal, political, social, or moral issues? How would that affect the pill addict who still suffers? How would it affect my own recovery?

7. At meetings, how do I feel when I hear someone share an opinion with which I strongly disagree? What could the speaker have done to change the way he expressed his opinion so that it would have bothered me less?

8. Which of my own opinions on outside issues have I shared at meetings? How did I express this information in a way that made it clear that these were only my opinions and did not represent the opinions of the group or of Pills Anonymous as a whole?

9. What outside issues have I developed very strong feelings about? Is it appropriate for me to share about these issues at meetings? If I do share about these issues, how can I do so without making other members uncomfortable?

10. What guidance has my sponsor offered about whether to share my ideas and opinions on these issues at meetings?

11. Do I always consider the effect of my words upon the unity of the group, or do I sometimes just share something to get it off my chest?

12. How can I use the underlying spiritual principles of the Tenth Tradition to minimize conflict in my personal life, as well as in Pills Anonymous?

TRADITION ELEVEN

"Our public relations policy is based on attraction rather than promotion; we need always maintain personal anonymity at the level of press, radio, television, and films."

To carry out our primary purpose of helping the pill addict who still suffers, we need to inform the general public of P.A.'s existence. The more the public knows about our fellowship and program, the more likely it is that pill addicts will think of us and try to find us when they want help.

We attempt to spread information about our program among the people most likely to come in contact with pill addicts, such as clergymen, medical professionals, law enforcement personnel, and social service organizations. We also try to inform members of the general public of our existence, so that the employers, friends, and families of pill addicts will be aware of us—and can reach us if they want more information. To increase the public's familiarity with Pills Anonymous, and to assist them in contacting us, we print announcements, participate in discussions in the media, write articles, publish and distribute books, make posters, create websites, and maintain phone lines. We attend health fairs and speak in classrooms, jails, hospitals, and other institutions. In short, we do everything we can to make ourselves widely recognized as an easily accessible organization dedicated to helping people recover from pill addiction.

This is such an important part of our mission that four of our twelve traditions deal exclusively with how our fellowship should present itself to the outside world. Tradition Six cautions us against endorsing, financing, or lending the P.A. name to other organizations, lest our fellowship become compromised or entangled. To further insure our integrity and independence, Tradition Seven encourages us to be fully self-supporting, declining all outside contributions. The Tenth Tradition advises P.A. to refrain from expressing opinions on outside issues so that our fellowship's name is never drawn into public controversy. Last, but certainly not least, Tradition Eleven defines our public relations policy as one of attraction rather than promotion, and advises us to observe personal anonymity when dealing with any media that might transmit information about our program.

For most of us, looking back on our own experience as newcomers is enough to convince us that it was attraction that drew us to P.A., not promotion. In the self-centeredness of our disease, many of us were manipulative people. We took advantage of our families, employers, and friends; and, most of all, we conned ourselves. In our self-delusion, we clung to the notion that there was nothing wrong with our pill use, until things finally got so bad that we were forced to seek help in the rooms of Pills Anonymous. Desperate and frightened, we skeptically listened to other pill addicts honestly share their experience, strength, and hope—and we eventually came to believe that if these people could learn to lead fulfilling lives without using pills, we could, too. Most of us were tired of all the lying and chaos that surrounded our pill use, and we were attracted to the honesty and serenity we found in many members of our fellowship. We responded to people who spoke truthfully, and who "walked the walk," confidently dealing with life on life's terms. We began to want what these people had to offer and became willing to try the program of Pills Anonymous in order to get it.

But how do we tell the difference between attraction and promotion? To do so, we must examine both the way in which the message is presented and the content of the message itself. We can understand the importance of presentation by asking ourselves how we would have responded to this program as newcomers if we had been lectured to, preached at, or assaulted with exaggerated claims. We can also look at how some of us carried the P.A. message in our early recovery. Our experience taught us that in spite of our good intentions, the louder we made our arguments, the less people tended to believe us. When we learn to present our message with honesty, simplicity, and humility, we find that we are more effective ambassadors for the P.A. program. As for the content of our message, we stick to simple, basic information. We explain what we do and where to find us. When we go beyond that, we risk crossing the line into promotion. Relying on our faith that the P.A. program works, we are able to deliver a simple, straightforward message, without fanfare, overblown claims, or celebrity endorsements.

The need for personal anonymity when dealing with the media is addressed in the second portion of the Eleventh Tradition. We have some latitude about identifying ourselves as members of P.A. to our family, friends, and co-workers, but we do not enjoy the same freedom when dealing with radio, TV, films, or any kind of printed media. In addition, although they are not specifically mentioned in the Eleventh Tradition, we apply the same standards when dealing with public internet venues such as social networking sites, forums, blogs, electronic bulletin boards, and the like. Although we do not divulge our last names or allow our faces to be photographed in connection with any public exposure involving Pills Anonymous, we are certainly not a secret society. As a matter of fact, our fellowship actively seeks ways to place itself in the public eye for the purpose of fulfilling our primary purpose, but the individual identities of our members should always be carefully hidden from public view.

We are vigilant about protecting the anonymity of our members so that people who have a pill problem will not be afraid to join us, and so that our current members continue to feel secure that their participation in this fellowship remains a confidential matter. If one of our members "goes public" in the media, it may give the false impression to newcomers that they, too, might have to reveal their identities in public. If one pill addict "outs" another in a public forum, either intentionally or unintentionally, still-suffering pill addicts may be reluctant to come to us for help, and pill addicts already in recovery may be tempted to leave. It is no exaggeration to say that lives could be lost as the result of such circumstances.

Our public relations policy of maintaining personal anonymity also protects P.A. as a whole from potential negative publicity. This becomes clear when we consider the potential dangers of encouraging celebrity endorsements. If someone famous publicly announces that they are a member of P.A., their personal opinions on any topic may be construed as representing the opinions of P.A. as a whole. And because they are closely scrutinized by the media, anything they say or do might result in our fellowship being found guilty by association.

Celebrity endorsements of our fellowship are a breach of both the promotion and anonymity portions of our Eleventh Tradition. Our members are free to publicly identify themselves as being "clean," "in a recovery program," or "having a sponsor," but when someone publicly says that they are a member of Pills Anonymous, they endanger the recovery of both potential and existing members. We cannot prevent celebrities or anyone else from publicly identifying themselves as members of our fellowship, but we can and should explain our Eleventh Tradition to the media, and ask them to refrain from publishing such information, although we cannot control whether they do so or not.

By breaking our personal anonymity in a public forum, we also jeopardize our own recovery. As pill addicts with super-sized egos, we have a tendency to emphasize how important we are as individuals. It comes as no surprise that many of us received poor grades in the "works and plays well with others" section of our report cards. Tradition Eleven helps to limit some of our behaviors that are based on the desire for personal recognition, power, prestige, and profit. This creates fewer problems for the fellowship, and for ourselves as well. It keeps the focus on the message, not the messenger. This is echoed by the principle of anonymity, which reminds us to always do what is right regardless of the individual personalities involved. There is a popular saying in our fellowship: "A pill addict alone is in bad company." This concept applies to our public relations efforts as well as to our personal recovery. By doing public information work in teams of two or more people, we help keep our individual personalities in check—and we also ensure that a single person is not representing the whole fellowship. Teamwork in public relations also fosters a spirit of unity, which is one of our fellowship's most appealing features—and one of its greatest strengths.

While the Eleventh Tradition specifically addresses our media relations, we can apply its principles to other forms of public relations in which all of our members play some part. We represent our fellowship when we wear a Pills Anonymous t-shirt, attend a group activity, or stand around talking after a meeting. In these situations, our behavior directly reflects on P.A., and should be a source of attraction, not embarrassment. When we are in the company of any non-member who is aware that we are in Pills Anonymous, we might want to remember that our words and demeanor form a living testament to the effectiveness of our program, and may encourage non-members to help spread the word about our fellowship. Ultimately, if we always bear in mind that our primary purpose is to carry a message of hope to the pill addict who still suffers, we will naturally become selfless and attractive representatives of Pills Anonymous.

OUR MEMBERS' EXPERIENCE WITH TRADITION ELEVEN

I GIVE MY VOICE TO MY HIGHER POWER

I have had mixed feelings about this tradition since coming to Pills Anonymous. With ever-increasing media coverage of the tragic effects of pill addiction, I often want to reach out, shout out, to let the media know about our fellowship. It seems that many media reports bombard us with the problem of pill addiction without offering information about viable solutions. Sadly, many still do not understand the nature of addiction. Twelve-step programs have worked for millions of people, and although there is no one proven way to stay clean, I wish the public could be given information about our way, a way that truly does work. I sometimes wonder, as more and more people suffer and die from pill addiction, why we can't get someone like a famous and well-respected talk-show host or doctor to spread the message of Pills Anonymous in a way that would reach millions with just one episode of their television show.

Yes, this would be a wonderful way to widely spread our message of hope for many. The problem is, who would be our spokesperson? To link a face and personality with Pills Anonymous would put our fellowship at risk for association with our spokesperson's beliefs, attitudes, and behaviors. No one is immune from being human, and human beings are fallible in ways big and small. Society can be ruthless and extremely critical of the smallest details, especially in their obsession with celebrities. In light of this, I understand that it would be dangerous to do anything less than maintain personal anonymity at the level of press, radio, television, and films.

What I *can* do to help spread the message of hope to others, is maintain an awareness of what I present to the world with my words, attitudes, and actions. I never know who might be watching my interactions or behavior and then show up later in a situation where I have the opportunity to be of service. If I am observed as being indifferent, rude, or dishonest, I may be presenting a negative image of Pills Anonymous and, therefore, have a poor chance of making a meaningful connection. On the other hand, when I live my life according to the spiritual principles of our program, living life centered in the present and respecting those around me, I have a good chance of attracting positive attention. I try to remember that I am a walking, talking representation of the quality of my recovery, my work with the Twelve Steps, and my connection with my Higher Power. When I am drawn into conversations about addiction, I give my voice to my Higher Power so that I am able to humbly and respectfully convey our message of recovery. Whatever the outcome, I believe my only job in such situations is to facilitate a bridge to recovery for the still-suffering addict. Today I know that no one even considers approaching that bridge if the entrance is not welcoming.

WORKING TRADITION ELEVEN

Tradition Eleven defines our public relations policy. Recognizing that the media is an important tool in furthering our primary purpose, this tradition sets forth guidelines for what we should say when publicly delivering the P.A. message. Answering these questions with the guidance of a sponsor may assist us in understanding the difference between attraction and promotion, and help us appreciate the importance of maintaining personal anonymity when representing P.A. in any public forum. Our answers may also help us to apply some of the underlying spiritual principles of the Eleventh Tradition in our daily lives, both inside and outside the rooms of Pills Anonymous.

1. In dealing with the media, what specific kinds of information about our program are appropriate to share? What are some examples of things that are <u>not</u> appropriate for us to discuss?

2. What is the difference between attraction and promotion? How do the spiritual principles of honesty and humility keep us from over-zealously "pitching" the benefits of P.A. to the public?

3. When I speak about our program to non-members or potential members of our fellowship, how can I stick to a simple message, instead of becoming "preachy"? What kinds of behavior or ways of presenting information might be interpreted as "preachy"? What are some of the possible consequences?

4. When I share at meetings, in what ways do I sometimes seek to attract attention to the messenger instead of the message? How can I correct this tendency?

5. What are some of the possible consequences of using our full names and/or photos when we identify ourselves in public as members of P.A.?

6. What are some of the possible consequences of celebrities publicly identifying themselves as members of Pills Anonymous? How might this publicity affect the celebrity himself, potential members, existing members, and P.A. as a whole?

7. How do our groups and service bodies ensure that no member has to do public information work alone?

8. How careful am I not to identify myself as a member of P.A. on social networking sites or other public internet forums? What can I do if another P.A. member breaks his own, someone else's, or my anonymity?

9. In what ways have I acted inappropriately in front of any non-members of P.A. who knew I was in the fellowship?

10. How can I use some of the underlying spiritual principles of the Eleventh Tradition, such as honesty, faith, humility, and integrity to help me in my personal relationships, and in other areas of my life?

TRADITION TWELVE

"Anonymity is the spiritual foundation of all our Traditions, ever reminding us to place principles before personalities."

Anonymity. It is hard to pronounce and even more difficult to practice. To be anonymous is to be of unknown origin or unnamed, as in "making an anonymous donation," or "quoting an anonymous source." And "anonymity" is simply the state of being anonymous. But what exactly does the "anonymous" in "Pills Anonymous" mean, and why is anonymity of such great importance to our fellowship?

At its most basic level, the practice of anonymity within our fellowship means not disclosing our full names or the full names of any other members. We withhold our last names so that existing or potential members, who are sometimes afraid their membership will become public knowledge, can participate in our fellowship without reservation. Practicing anonymity at this level provides a safe environment for our members, allowing them to openly and honestly share their experiences without fear of being publicly exposed. Pill addicts might hesitate to turn to P.A. for help if they thought their privacy might be invaded, or if there was a risk that their problems might become known outside of our meetings. We always try to remind each other that everything we see and hear at our meetings should stay there. We try to avoid using our full names during meetings, at P.A. events, and if possible, when conducting P.A. business. At times it may be necessary or even advisable to share our last names with fellow members, or to say that we are members of P.A. to non-members or potential members, but not if such an act needlessly jeopardizes the sense of security we try to cultivate for the members of our fellowship.

The wording of Tradition Twelve also suggests a much broader interpretation of the word "anonymity." At the root of our disease is self-will, and in our individual recovery, we seek to replace this self-will with the guidance of a Higher Power of our own understanding. When we embark upon the Twelve Steps, we first admit that we are powerless, then come to believe that a power greater than ourselves can restore us to sanity, and finally, we turn our will and our lives over to the care of God as we understand Him. Our Twelfth Tradition applies this same process of surrender to the way we work together as a fellowship. It suggests that we humbly put our personal desires aside and surrender our self-will to the collective conscience of the group, whose ultimate authority is a loving God. This surrender for the good of the fellowship is the deeper, spiritual meaning of anonymity, a definition that firmly establishes it as the spiritual foundation of all twelve of our traditions.

Our First Tradition helps to keep our individual egos in check by placing our common welfare above our individual interest. Being anonymous by surrendering our self-will, P.A. unity becomes our number one priority, because without it we would have no P.A. fellowship to foster our own individual recovery. Anonymity is also at the heart of Tradition Two, which advises us that our groups should accept only one ultimate authority—a loving God as He may express Himself in our group conscience. Our leaders are asked to humbly accept the anonymity of their positions as servants, not governors. In this context, anonymity means we are each just one among many, with no single person any more or less important than anyone else in the fellowship.

Tradition Three fosters anonymity by establishing the desire to stop using pills as the sole requirement for membership. This creates a strong bond of equality among us, enabling us to set aside our sometimes vast personal differences so that we can help each other with our common problem. Tradition Four applies the principle of anonymity to our groups. Every P.A. group has an equal place in our fellowship, with equal rights and responsibilities, and each group is free to act independently, according to its own group conscience, except in matters affecting other groups or P.A. as a whole. By practicing anonymity at the group level, we encourage a spirit of cooperation, not competition. The Fifth Tradition reinforces the principle of anonymity by supplying our groups with a clear, uncomplicated mission statement—to carry the message of recovery to the pill addict who still suffers. As long as we maintain our focus on the primary purpose of our fellowship, we can avoid acting on our own individual, egotistical agendas.

The principle of anonymity also shapes our fellowship's dealings with society at large. Our Sixth Tradition reminds us that P.A. should never allow its name to be used by another organization, and that P.A. should not use any other organization's name to advance our fellowship. In principle, our relationships with the outside world are forged through the thoughtful and unified collective conscience of our groups, and do not depend on the diverse individual personalities of our members. Anonymity also inspires our principle of service rotation, which helps to make our representatives and leaders interchangeable, and therefore, anonymous. This assists our fellowship in avoiding the pitfalls of money, property, and prestige that might divert us from our primary purpose. Our groups depend on the Seventh Tradition to keep our funding (and the financing of the entire fellowship) anonymous. We simply pass a basket at meetings, and do not keep track of how much each member contributes. Our groups are encouraged to depend on all of their members equally, which allows selfless giving to flourish side by side with collective, anonymous responsibility.

Selfless anonymity is also the cornerstone of Tradition Eight. All of our members are equally qualified to carry the message of recovery to other pill addicts, and are expected to do so without any expectation of reward or recognition. We do our best to avoid profiting financially from our service to the fellowship, and we shun personal acclaim by drawing attention to the message, not the messenger. Our service bodies, as defined by Tradition Nine, protect our anonymity by ensuring that one member never becomes more important than any other. As frequently as is practical, our service positions are rotated among our members, and by keeping our service boards and committees strictly accountable to the groups they serve, we ensure that individuals in service do not act independently.

To properly observe our Tenth Tradition we must accept and put into practice the principle of anonymity. It is fine for us to be opinionated as individuals, but when representing Pills Anonymous, we refrain from expressing our personal opinions so that our fellowship is kept free from controversy. Tradition Eleven steers us to a public relations policy based on attraction rather than promotion, and encourages us to restrain our egos so that we can present our message in a simple, straightforward way, without fanfare or exaggeration. The Eleventh Tradition also stresses the importance of maintaining personal anonymity in all public media. "Anonymity" also means "faceless," so whenever there is a direct public connection with the fellowship of Pills Anonymous, we withhold our full names, and also do all we can to prevent the publication of images that identify members of our fellowship, whether they are celebrities or not.

Observance of the Twelfth Tradition depends on the humility that results from working the Twelve Steps, which are the antidote for the arrogant self-centeredness we developed as pill addicts. As we mature in our recovery, we begin to accept responsibility for our actions and allow a Higher Power to relieve us of some of our shortcomings. Our behavior gradually changes. We no longer try to elevate ourselves by belittling others or "stealing the show." We stop insisting on having our own way. We no longer have to believe or pretend that we know more than others, and we stop trying to "fix" other people or situations. In short, we humbly surrender control of our lives and the lives of others to a Higher Power of our own individual understanding.

We are forced to call upon this newfound humility when we begin working on the Twelfth Step, gratefully carrying the message to pill addicts and practicing the spiritual principles of the Twelve Steps in all our affairs. Consciously or unconsciously, as we progress along this path, we begin to accept the Twelfth Tradition and the principle of anonymity. The more we unselfishly engage in service to the fellowship, the more "I" becomes "we," and the better we feel about ourselves as we become part of a greater whole. When we honestly seek the group's success rather than our own, we naturally place the spiritual principles of the Twelve Traditions above the opinions of individual personalities. By placing principles before personalities, we avoid disrupting our fellowship with our egotistical behavior, and we are able to resolve differences that sometimes arise with other members. The spiritual spark that was almost extinguished by our disease is re-ignited by our selfless, anonymous service, and we are rewarded with continued recovery, and a sense of satisfaction and fulfillment that exceeds even our greatest expectations.

OUR MEMBERS' EXPERIENCE
WITH TRADITION TWELVE

MY EGO IS A TYRANT

One of the definitions of the word "anonymous" is "lacking individuality, unique character, or distinction." One of the problems I had during my first two rounds with recovery was that I thought I was unique. Yes, my substance abuse had gotten the best of me. I had earned a place in outpatient and inpatient treatment programs, but after those short stints of acquiring knowledge and proving I could stay drug-free, I thought I was better. I had not reached the same levels of despair and destruction as others in treatment. After a round of rehab, I rationalized that I had all I needed and my head was back on straight, so I moved on and wished good luck to all those who *truly* had a problem. It was not until my affair with pills nearly buried me that I surrendered my "uniqueness" and sought true recovery in the rooms of Pills Anonymous. I have come to learn and realize with ever-increasing awareness that many of my problems centered on ego. My ego is a tyrant that, if pacified and allowed to rule, will twist, damage, and destroy any and all situations and relationships to serve its desires. My ego separates me from my fellows and tells me that I am special and not like everyone else. For this pill addict, and for the fellowship as a whole, anonymity protects me—and our fellowship—from the effects of ego.

One of the first meetings I attended was in the inner city of a large metropolitan area. The neighborhood was old and run-down. As I approached the building, I thought that the people standing outside looked a bit rough. I went to the meeting alone, a female still shaky from withdrawal and feeling very vulnerable. I had made a commitment to attend meetings and I was serious about following through, but when the people standing outside noticed me and looked my way, I was really scared. All I wanted to do was turn and run, yet from out of nowhere a voice in my head said, "principles before personalities, principles before personalities," and I kept walking. I made it into the building and took a seat. I felt terribly conspicuous. I looked like a rainbow-colored lollipop amidst a sea of black leather and denim, but I managed to muster the courage to raise my hand when they asked if there were any newcomers. What totally blew me away after the meeting ended was the warmth and love given to me by those "rough people" whose personalities I had judged and feared based on my impression of their appearance. I was not different and I was not special or out of place. I was just another suffering addict looking for a solution. Every woman in that room looked past my personality and employed the principles of our program by reaching out and offering me experience, strength, and hope. They also passed around a meeting list and wrote their phone numbers on it for me.

It turned out that I learned a powerful lesson about the principles of recovery that day. I remember this experience and I do my best to remember the damage my ego can do if I allow it to edge out the principles I have learned in Pills Anonymous. Love, tolerance, acceptance, humility, surrender, and perseverance are but a few that help keep me grounded and centered.

WORKING TRADITION TWELVE

Observing Tradition Twelve is critical when doing service work of any kind. Service work means helping to carry the message of Pills Anonymous in any one of many different ways. And in keeping with the principle of anonymity, no service or servant is more important than any other. Making coffee before the meeting or greeting newcomers; participating in a panel at a local recovery

center, or serving as our group's secretary or treasurer; partici-
pating in service at the area, regional, or world level; presenting
information about P.A. publicly or to the media; cleaning up after
a meeting, or even just showing up, are all equally important ways
in which we can express our gratitude and carry the message. We
keep what we have by giving it away, but how we give it away is
also of great importance. Answering these questions can help us to
understand and apply the Twelfth Tradition in service work and in
our personal lives as well.

1. What have I done in the past, and what am I doing today to help fulfill P.A.'s primary purpose?

2. How important is my service work to the success of P.A.?

3. How important is service work to my own recovery? Why and how do we thank our fellow members for letting us be of service?

4. Why is it important that I perform my service in accordance with all of our traditions, especially the Twelfth Tradition? How can I be sure that I am performing my service in this way?

5. What are some of the possible consequences of breaking my own anonymity, or that of other P.A. members?

6. For most of us, there have been occasions when we felt it was appropriate to reveal our membership in Pills Anonymous to non-members or potential members. What consideration did I give to the principle of anonymity, and to the advice of my sponsor when I made this decision?

7. How much pride do I feel when I put money in the basket, and how much superiority or resentment do I feel when I put money in and others do not? Why is it

important for our financial contributions to P.A. to be anonymous?

8. Why is humility so important to the principle of anonymity?

9. In what ways do I call attention to myself when I am sharing or doing service work of any kind? How can I become less egocentric and more selfless?

10. How much importance do I attach to what my fellow P.A. members think of me? In what ways is this healthy, and in what ways is it unhealthy?

11. What is the meaning of the expression, "learning to separate the people from the problem," and how does it relate to placing principles before personalities?

12. In what ways have the lessons of the Twelfth Tradition helped me in my everyday life, especially in my relationships with family and friends, and at school, work, or in other organizations with which I am involved?

THE IMPORTANCE OF "ANONYMITY"

Traditionally, P.A. members take great care to preserve their anonymity at the public level: press, radio, television and films. We know from experience that people with drug problems might hesitate to turn to P.A. for help if they thought their problems might be discussed publicly, even inadvertently, by others. Newcomers should be able to seek help with complete assurance that their identities will not be disclosed to anyone outside the Fellowship.

We believe that the concept of personal anonymity has a spiritual significance for us: it discourages the drives for personal recognition, power, prestige, or profit that have caused difficulties in some societies. Much of our relative effectiveness in working with addicts might be impaired if we sought or accepted public recognition.

While each member of P.A. is free to make his or her own interpretation of P.A. Tradition, no individual is ever recognized as a spokesperson for the Fellowship locally, nationally or internationally. Each member speaks only for themselves. Pills Anonymous is grateful to all media for their assistance in strengthening and observing the Tradition of anonymity.

Periodically, the P.A. World Service Office may send to all major media a letter describing the Traditions and asking their support in observing it.

A P.A. member may, for various reasons, "break anonymity" deliberately at the public level. Since that is a matter of individual choice and conscience, the Fellowship as a whole has no control over such deviations from Tradition. It is clear, however, that they do not have the approval of the group conscience of P.A. members.

P.A. Definition of Clean Time and Recovery

In Pills Anonymous, we believe clean time is based on abstinence from pills and all other mind-altering substances. Many of us came to P.A. due to addiction to prescribed medications, but we believe abstinence should NOT be limited to pills alone. As addicts we say that we have given up our right to seek a "sense of ease and comfort" from ALL mind-altering substances including, but not limited to: certain prescribed medications, alcohol, street drugs, and even some over-the-counter medications.

We understand there are instances in which mind-altering medication may be necessary. We suggest when these circumstances arise, we inform our doctors of our recovery from pill addiction, speak with our sponsor, and share our situation with other members of P.A. before making a decision about taking such medication.

Recovery is our goal, not just physical abstinence. We have found that through the P.A program our perception has changed and we no longer see using pills as the solution. We believe the best foundation for maintaining and enjoying recovery is through sharing our experience, strength, and hope with each other and by working the Twelve Steps of Pills Anonymous.

Made.in the USA
Monee, IL
15 May 2020